MIND

BODY

BUMP

BRIT WILLIAMS

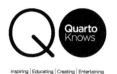

Brimming with creative inspiration, how-to projects, and useful information to enrich your everyday life, Quarto Knows is a favourite destination for those pursuing their interests and passions. Visit our site and dig deeper with our books into your area of interest: Quarto Creates, Quarto Cooks, Quarto Homes, Quarto Lives, Quarto Drives, Quarto Explores, Quarto Gifts, or Quarto Kids.

First published in 2019 by White Lion Publishing,
an imprint of The Quarto Group.
The Old Brewery, 6 Blundell Street
London, N7 9BH,
United Kingdom
T (0)20 7700 6700
www.QuartoKnows.com

A catalogue record for this book is available from the British Library.

ISBN 978 1 78131 858 4
Ebook ISBN 978 1 78131 859 1

10 9 8 7 6 5 4 3 2 1

Design by Gemma Wilson
Photography by Simon Pask, with the exception of pages 59, 83, 119, 171 © Mindful Chef; 72, 122 © Sophie Keogh @sophiemarielouisek; 174 © Mona Godfrey
Illustrations by Lizzy Thomas
Medical read by Dr Maggie Blott

Printed in China

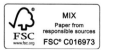

MIND BODY BUMP

THE COMPLETE PLAN FOR AN ACTIVE PREGNANCY

BRIT WILLIAMS

INCLUDES
RECIPES BY

Mindful
Chef

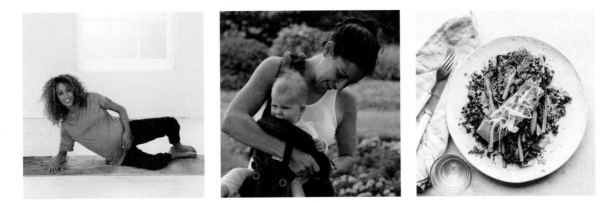

WITH FOREWORD BY TAMARA HILL-NORTON, SWEATY BETTY FOUNDER

Contents

Foreword

What a brilliant book for expectant mums! If you have enjoyed training – especially strength training – before your pregnancy, *Mind, Body, Bump* will be an insightful and inspiring support as you transition to training for two.

I wish I'd had Brit's book on my shelf during my three pregnancies. In the early 2000s, there was nothing like this for prenatal women. I remember well how people would tell me I shouldn't be raising my heart rate and how I should do little more than some gentle prenatal yoga. Without much information available, I didn't know who or what to believe; aside from cycling and yoga, I prevented myself from doing the exercise I loved best.

The other experience I remember poignantly is the guilt when I did carve out time to train. During my last pregnancy I had weekly sessions with a prenatal trainer, but it entailed leaving my home and my children on top of taking time away from family to run my business. For busy mums-to-be and mums with younger children, I particularly love the flexibility and adaptability of Brit's programme. You can work out at home and spend as long or little as you can, all while knowing you are receiving the best advice and guidance.

Having worked with Brit and watched her journey through personal training and motherhood, I cannot imagine a more passionate and qualified trainer to be there for every step of your active pregnancy. You can hear her enthusiasm in the way she writes. She includes all the information you could ever want, but makes it accessible with personal anecdotes and a sense of humour that reminds us that exercise is a fun and enjoyable part of pregnancy. *Mind, Body, Bump* is the next best thing to having Brit there by your side.

There is a lot of synergy between *MBB* and Sweaty Betty. Our mission is to empower women through fitness and beyond, and Brit is supporting that empowerment through one precious and incomparably rewarding female experience. I wish you well on your *MBB* journey, and hope that pregnancy and motherhood enables you to become your strongest, happiest self yet.

Tamara
FOUNDER & CHIEF CREATIVE OFFICER OF SWEATY BETTY

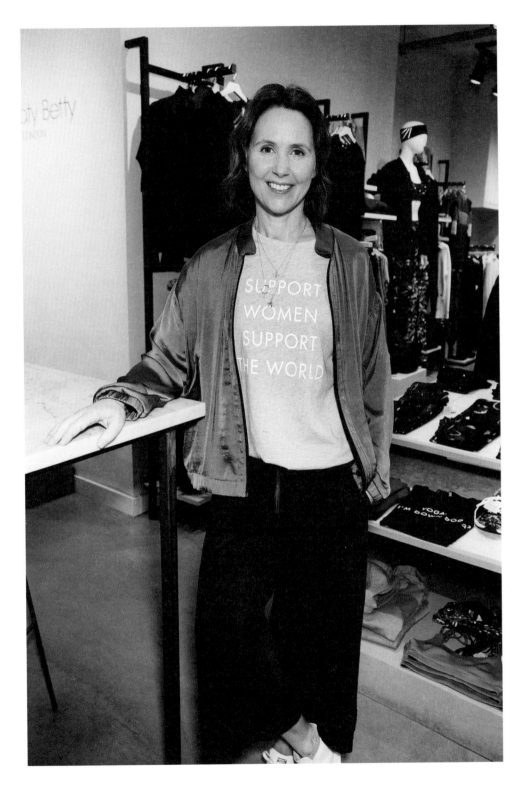

The Birth of
Mind, Body, Bump

There are a handful of experiences in life that leave you wondering how you got from 'there' to 'here'. Pregnancy is one of them. Becoming a mother is, perhaps, the biggest one of all. For me, writing this book has been another. It is fitting, then, that I've filled the following pages during the first six months of getting to know my daughter, and that, in becoming a mother, I've had the opportunity to reflect on the unique 'there-ness' of pregnancy.

At every turn of pregnancy – from the moment the stick turns blue to the first scan, the emergence of your bump to the initial exhilarating contraction – there is a sense of leaping suddenly and irreversibly away from the familiar comfort of 'there' and arriving at a kind of limbo that we can only describe as 'here'.

Pregnancy is arguably nature's most transient phenomenon. Among its rapid physical and mental changes, the only real continuity is a sense of waiting . . . and waiting . . .

The word itself implies inactivity, awkward stillness and uncertainty, but this doesn't have to be the case. Life needn't stop when you're expecting. It's just beginning – in more ways than one. This book explores how to stop waiting and start living, by embracing action and reclaiming ownership over the 'here', wherever 'here' is for you.

Exercise is an opportunity to quiet a busy **mind** and focus on the simplicity of moving and breathing. Each workout improves your physical awareness, while achievements along the way help you to celebrate your changing **body**. Let's not forget about the source of change – the beautiful baby growing beneath your **bump**. It makes good sense that the healthier your body, the healthier the baby who calls it home.

Mind, Body, Bump is the result of trialing hundreds of exercises while pregnant myself, as well as creating and modifying prenatal training plans for many expectant mums, who have since given birth to thriving babies and continued to enjoy exercise as new mums. Throughout the book I'll refer to modifications as 'pregnancy-progressive'. Some of these modifications may not look like the 'progressions' you're used to in workouts, such as moving faster or lifting heavier, but they're adapted to benefit your body from one phase of pregnancy to the next. After all, you're producing a tiny miracle inside you, and there's no denying that's a pretty progressive task.

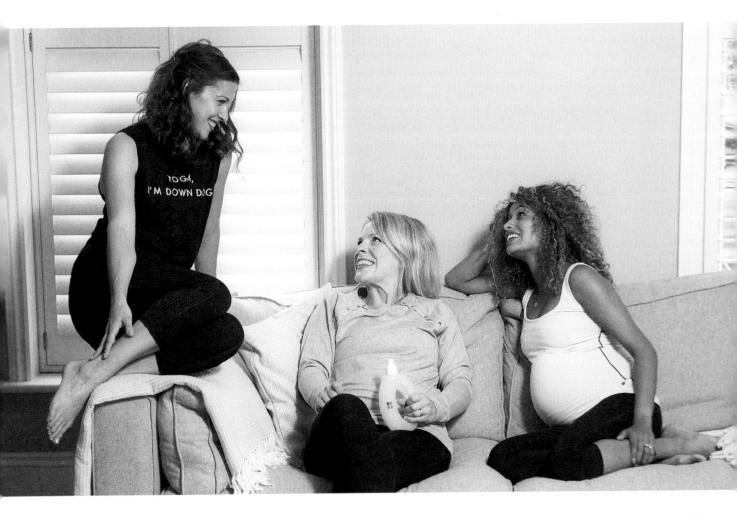

The Benefits of Exercising in Pregnancy

The most inspiring evidence for staying active is the example set by exceptional athletes who have continued to train and compete throughout their pregnancies. Most recently, Serena Williams has been hailed the mother of all athletes, winning the 2017 Australian Open while pregnant and returning to Wimbledon within a year of the birth of her daughter. British Ultra Runner Sophie Power also proved mothers can go the distance during the 166km Ultra Trail Mont Blanc in 2018, which she successfully completed while expressing milk and breastfeeding her three-month-old baby boy. Sophie gives her pre-natal training full credit for her strong recovery, and found that her labour was easier for being fitter.

Beyond providing a means of carving out valuable you-time during pregnancy, exercise has ample benefits for both you and your growing baby. Listen to your body and seek out any action that creates a health- and happiness-boosting reaction.

Recent studies have invalidated old fears about prenatal exercise, instead proving that an active pregnancy can aid fetal heart health, reduce maternal hypertension and support a shorter labour. Training can also improve lower-back strength and reduce pregnancy-related injuries. University of Montreal researchers have even identified a positive link between active pregnancies and advanced neurodevelopment in newborns – yet more evidence that workouts are physically and mentally beneficial for expectant mums and their babies.

The science is compelling. But there's one benefit of prenatal exercise that is even more obvious: it makes you feel good.

I'm not just talking about feel-good endorphins, which will undoubtedly give you a buzz that turns any waddle into serious pregnancy swag. A consistent prenatal training programme achieves far-reaching benefits, buckling you into the driving seat during the wild ride of pregnancy. The focus required during the more technical aspects of strength training in particular encourages you to turn your mind inwards and manifest the kind of self-belief that helps to frame pregnancy and labour in a positive light.

Television presenter, mother and fitness expert Davina McCall brilliantly stated that 'fear is the greatest closer of cervixes'. I couldn't agree more, which is why the benefits of this book exceed the physical benefits of working out. The same self-belief that gets you through your workouts will guide you calmly and confidently through your labour. You'll discover strength you didn't know you had, tap into newfound respect for your body and connect deeply and meaningfully to your baby. You're about to undertake the ultimate labour of love.

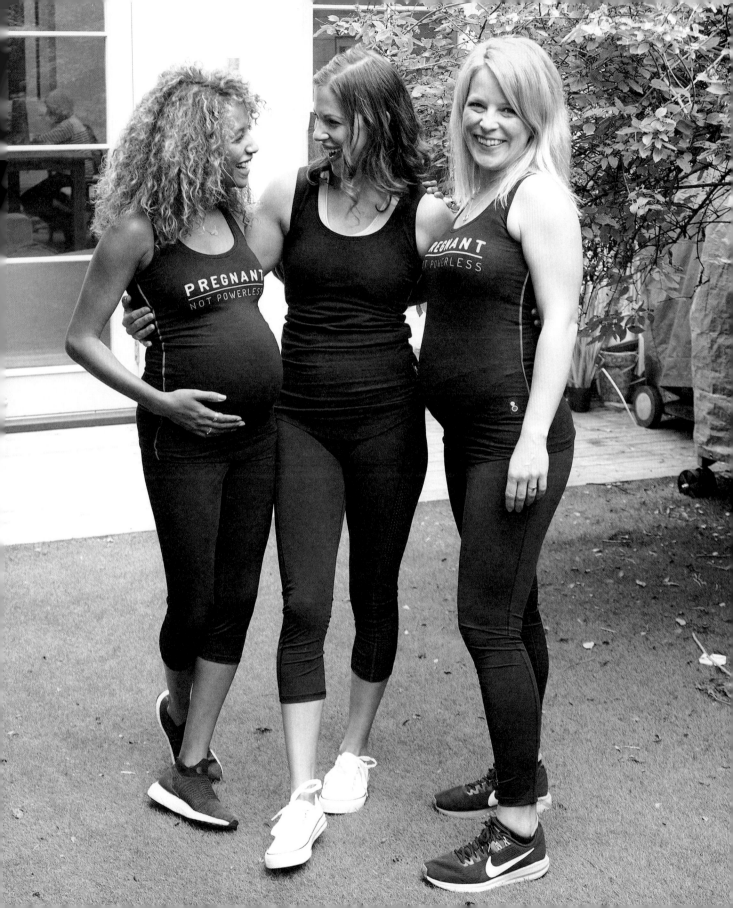

Your Unique Journey

If you are diagnosed with any of the following conditions during your pregnancy, they could mean that you should avoid particular exercises. Speak to your doctor or midwives about how best to manage your condition and remain active.

- Low-lying placenta
- Hypertension
- Anaemia
- Chronic bronchitis
- Gestational diabetes
- Fetal growth restriction
- Weak cervix

There are highlights and challenges of pregnancy that everyone is likely to encounter at some point. The excitement, maternal glow and baby kicks on one hand; the nausea, fatigue and physical aches on the other. The frequency and intensity of these highs and lows varies significantly from person to person, and indeed from pregnancy to pregnancy. Whatever your ambitions for keeping active during pregnancy, please avoid comparing yourself to anyone else – or even to yourself, if you've been here before.

The workouts in this book act as a guide to make you feel safe and strong when you train, but it is impossible to account for every sensation you may feel throughout your pregnancy. During personal training sessions, I use the warm-up to get a sense of how my clients are feeling and moving. There are a myriad of changes that will, and should, influence your training. For that reason, I ask you to never skip your warm-up. This is the most important time to internalise your awareness and make important decisions about what you need from your training from one day to the next.

Your best coach along the way will invariably be your own body. Learn to listen to it.

While exercise offers a way for you to feel empowered and take control of your pregnancy, it's important to defer to your doctor if you have any doubt about your own well-being or that of your baby. If you experience any of the following symptoms during exercise, stop immediately and consult a doctor. There's probably a very simple explanation, but peace of mind is a priority when you're training for two.

WHEN TO STOP EXERCISE

- Vaginal bleeding
- Dizziness
- Shortness of breath
- Severe headache
- Abdominal pain
- Chest pain or palpitations
- Substantial swelling in face, hands or legs
- Decreased fetal movement
- Leaking amniotic fluid
- Significant and sustained back pain

Perhaps the best thing you can do to support your pregnancy is to celebrate your body for what it has achieved. *Mind, Body, Bump* does just that. It celebrates your body by preserving and enhancing its ability to support you every step of the way. It also incorporates mindfulness techniques, encouraging you to feel specific muscles awaken and to use the breath as you move. As you become more aware of your body, you can also be more mentally present in your workout. You'll learn transferable skills that support you long after your cool-down, helping you to live positively in the moment rather than anxiously in a world of 'what ifs'.

EXERCISING THROUGH FERTILITY TREATMENT

Moderate exercise is almost always beneficial for fertility. However, frequent vigorous exercise can cause unhelpful physical stress. If you are looking to become pregnant through fertility treatment, take advice from your consultants about how best to support each phase. There may be days when the hormonal effects of treatment leave you feeling drained, in which case the best thing you can do is rest.

When you do feel energetic enough to exercise, be confident in the fact that the workouts in this book are designed to challenge your body without putting undue stress on your baby. They are also low impact and modifiable, so you can approach them differently according to how you feel.

An Active Pregnancy

You have already read how beneficial keeping active can be for you and your developing baby. Most health organisations recommend at least 120 minutes of moderate exercise every week throughout pregnancy. Alongside the workouts in this book, a host of other activities offer great support for expectant mums. Walking, swimming and dedicated prenatal Pilates and yoga classes are fantastic resources to keep you and bump moving.

If you are a keen runner or cyclist, you can continue to enjoy these activities for much of your pregnancy with just a few sensible precautions. Excess impact can weaken the pelvic floor, so I recommend swapping your high-energy runs for vigorous hikes after month five. Take care to cycle in a way that reduces any chance of a fall or collision – ideally on designated lanes and trails with which you're familiar. Remember that your balance will be affected as your bump grows. Consider swapping to indoor stationary cycling in the second half of your pregnancy, which is a great tool for scaling the intensity of your workouts, and allows you to assume a more comfortable upright position.

Resistance training – particularly when performed in circuits that keep your heart rate safely elevated – offers another way to maintain your fitness, with the added benefit of strengthening specific muscles that weaken during pregnancy.

TRAINING FOR A HEALTHY PREGNANCY

Although the physical changes of pregnancy are numerous, the major transitions are predictable. For that reason, we can train in ways that look ahead, to prevent or reduce uncomfortable symptoms rather than reacting to symptoms as they appear.

Here are four common prenatal symptoms and how you can stay one step ahead of them:

PELVIC PAIN This usually kicks in during the second and third trimesters. Reduce impact activities and modify your range of movement as necessary to ease downward pressure.

BACK PAIN AND SCIATICA Strengthen supporting glute and anterior core muscles with exercises like bridges and deadlifts to minimise strain on the lumbar spine.

HYPERMOBILE JOINTS Safely load the supporting muscles of the shoulders, hips and knees with manageable yet challenging weights to optimise muscle tone. Full body exercises like squat thrusters will build strength and stability in all three.

OVERACTIVE HIP FLEXORS Maintain core strength and optimise glute strength in order to minimise overcompensation by the hip flexors as your bump grows.

Most aches and pains during pregnancy result from muscular imbalances. You can avoid developing these by choosing exercises that condition the muscles that will come under most strain. This includes the upper and lower back, core, hamstrings and glutes. While a strong core is important to support your growing bump, pregnancy is not the time to overexert the abdominals with crunching movements. We'll explore plenty of safe and beneficial ways to optimise your core strength without a single crunch.

This book supports you through each trimester, explaining the modifications needed to keep you exercising safely at each stage. The one variable of exercise you should observe throughout your pregnancy is *intensity*. You can moderate intensity by playing with pace, range of movement and weight selection. A working rate of exertion (RPE) of around 8/10 will help you maximise the benefits of exercise without overworking. An easy measure of this is that you should be able to talk while you train. Take care that your range of movement and level of impact are also kind to your joints, which are less stable and more prone to hyperflexibility at this time.

Nourish for Two

Your body needs quality nutrition in order to perform well in training and to recover well outside of training. When you're sharing your nutrients with a growing baby, this is truer than ever.

Firstly, let's replace the concept of eating for two with one of nourishing for two. Although I recommend listening to your body and not obsessing over calorie intake, it's useful to know that caloric demand doesn't actually increase until the third trimester. Even then, the additional requirement is around 300 calories – the equivalent of a light snack. Prioritise quality in the form of a balanced and varied diet over a higher quantity of less nutrient-dense foods.

Throughout my pregnancy I considered how the food I ate served my nutritional goals. Focusing on the benefits of what you eat helps you feel happy and positive about food, which I firmly believe is best served with enjoyment. Here are a few simple guidelines for a healthy, obsession-free prenatal diet:

OPTIMISE YOUR ENERGY LEVELS Eat four to six small daily meals that include a roughly even balance of carbohydrates, protein and healthy fats to stabilise blood sugar.

NOURISH YOUR CELLS Refuel after exercise and tackle the extra cellular wear-and-tear of pregnancy by incorporating quality proteins and wholegrains, which help to rebuild tissue.

TOP UP ON MIGHTY MINERALS The easiest way to ensure you get the whole spectrum of vitamins and essential minerals – such as iron, calcium and magnesium – is to include a rainbow of fruit and vegetables in your daily diet.

SUPPLEMENT WISELY Choose a high-quality prenatal supplement which includes 400mcg folic acid and 10mcg vitamin D – both essential for your baby's brain, spinal cord and skeletal development.

AVOID POTENTIAL TOXINS Some foods carry a higher risk of salmonella, listeria, toxoplasmosis and mineral toxicity. Refer to the panel on which foods to avoid, and consider choosing organic produce to reduce exposure to pesticides.

VEGETARIAN AND VEGAN PREGNANCIES

If you are vegetarian, there are a few pregnancy-specific demands that require mindful ingredient selection or additional supplementation. Try to eat as many plant-based complete proteins as possible, including soy, quinoa, buckwheat, spirulina, chorella and amaranth. You can also mix two sources of incomplete protein – including grains, nuts and legumes – to provide all nine essential amino acids in a single meal. If you don't eat fish, it's recommended you take an algae-based omega-3 supplement. Vegetarians can also be more prone to anaemia – particularly during pregnancy – so regularly top up on plant-based iron sources, including leafy greens, beetroot, lentils and nuts.

Many vitamins and minerals prevalent in meat and fish can be found in eggs or dairy instead. If you are vegan, you may struggle to get sufficient B12, which works alongside folic acid to form baby's DNA and support fetal brain development. Speak to a qualified nutritionist as early as possible to discuss an appropriate B12 supplement. If you avoid dairy, look to green leafy veg and superfood chia seeds to up your plant-based calcium intake. This will aid baby's skeletal development through the first two trimesters and support muscle contractions during labour. Finally, look to seaweeds as a dairy-free, plant-based source of iodine, which is essential for fetal brain development.

THE RECIPES IN THIS BOOK

As nutrition is so essential to a healthy, active pregnancy, I am thrilled to partner with Mindful Chef – a London-based farm-to-table food delivery brand. They have provided mouthwatering meat and plant-based recipes to inspire your mealtimes and support the prenatal body. I hope they renew your love for quality nutrition and fine flavour as you nourish for two.

FOODS TO AVOID IN PREGNANCY

- Soft unpasteurised cheese such as brie, camembert, goat's cheese, blue cheese
- Unpasteurised dairy
- Undercooked eggs
- Paté
- Undercooked or cured meats
- Liver
- Game
- Shark, swordfish or marlin
- Raw shellfish
- Unfrozen sushi or unfarmed fresh salmon sushi
- Alcohol
- Caffeine in excess of 200mg per day

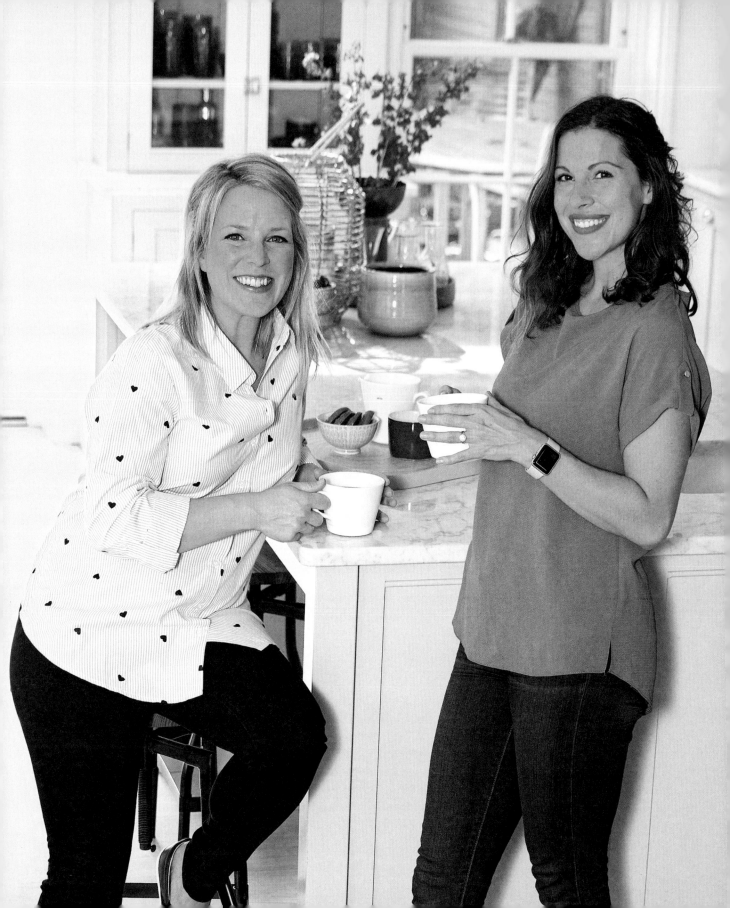

Friends, Family and Partner

Whether I was supporting clients or undertaking my own workout, I spent a lot my pregnancy at the squat rack. I'm lucky that I work within a supportive community, and generally everyone cheered me on as my bump grew bigger and I continued to weight train.

I've spoken to women who haven't felt their prenatal fitness efforts were so well understood. Although we have science on our side (and, more importantly, millions of healthy babies born out of active pregnancies), outdated custom and language can put unnecessary limitations on expectant mothers.

The best way to encounter naysayers is to be armed with knowledge, of which I hope you'll find plenty within these pages. If sceptics can understand your motivation – to strengthen your body for the physical changes of pregnancy, to promote optimal health for you and your baby, to improve your mental well-being and to enhance your labour experience and facilitate a safe postpartum recovery – there is little to which they can object.

A great way to celebrate your active pregnancy is to share it with others. If you have other children, go to the pool as a family at the weekends. Share the language of this book with your partner – such as building a baby athlete and hitting baby personal bests (PBs) – so you can acknowledge your prenatal fitness milestones together. If it's important to you that exercise is time for yourself, reassure friends and family that you're training for mental well-being and that your workouts allow you to communicate better and enjoy greater quality of time together.

I hope too that *MBB* gives you a sense of wider support and community. In writing this book, it is my intention to enable a shift towards prenatal fitness dialogue that's centred around what women can do rather than what they can't. To do that, I also ask you to pass the baton. I encourage you to connect with others in person and online, share your #mindbodybump progress and help to frame prenatal training as an exercise in self-belief for expectant mothers. Still a new mum as I fill these pages, I know now more than ever that victory is greatest when achieved hand in hand.

How to Use This Book

The *Mind, Body, Bump* workouts suggest ways in which you can stay challenged and excited about exercise while protecting your prenatal body (and its precious cargo). You can follow them to the letter, or you can adapt them to suit your body, resources and lifestyle.

Each month includes two new workouts – one bodyweight session and one resistance-based session – designed to complement that specific stage of pregnancy. Month one introduces some foundational movements that you will come back to and modify throughout your pregnancy. That's why, even if you're beginning the workouts after your first month of pregnancy, I suggest working through these early routines at least a couple times before moving onto subsequent months.

Each workout provides recommendations to suit two levels of fitness – Mindful Mamas and Tandem Athletes. Use your pre-pregnancy fitness level to decide which recommendations to follow. If you regularly participated in weight training before pregnancy and you're familiar with the movements in the workout, you will probably excel with the Tandem Athlete instructions. If you're new to weight-based training or building your confidence in compound movements such as squats and deadlifts, start with the Mindful Mama suggestions and consider progressing to Tandem Athlete if you require a greater challenge. If you have no equipment but still want to try the workouts, you also have the option to follow only the bodyweight sessions.

For the best results, I recommend doing each workout at least once a week and supplementing with an additional cardio-focused workout. Choose an activity in which you're already proficient. If you are a runner, I suggest swapping jogging for hiking, stationary cycling, swimming or other low-impact aerobics after month five. If you are able to incorporate three workouts per week, double up on the bodyweight workout one week, then on the resistance-based workout the next. Always choose the type and intensity of your prenatal workouts based on your confidence in those activities before pregnancy. This is a time to continue the training you love rather than dabble in drastically new forms of exercise.

Most importantly, enjoy and celebrate your body!

EQUIPMENT

Staying active during pregnancy doesn't require an expensive gym membership or endless free time. All the workouts are designed to take less than an hour and to use your own body weight or versatile resistance equipment that you can store at home.

For the resistance workouts, you will require the following:

One medium kettlebell between 6–10kg (13–22lb), or one light (4–8kg/9–18lb) and one heavy (8–12kg/18–26lb) at either end of the spectrum

One pair of light to medium dumbbells between 3–6kg (7–13lb), two pairs at either end of the spectrum or a set of adaptable dumbbell bars and weight plates

One light to medium resistance band, ideally with handles

One medium to strong resistance loop

One set of gliders, ideally double-sided for suitability on hard and carpeted floors

One high-quality exercise mat (non-essential but useful for all exercises)

One Swiss ball

One aerobic step (third trimester only)

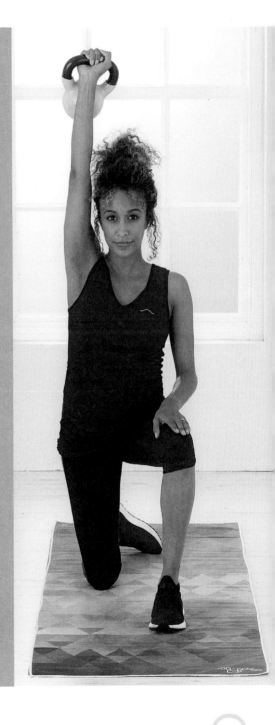

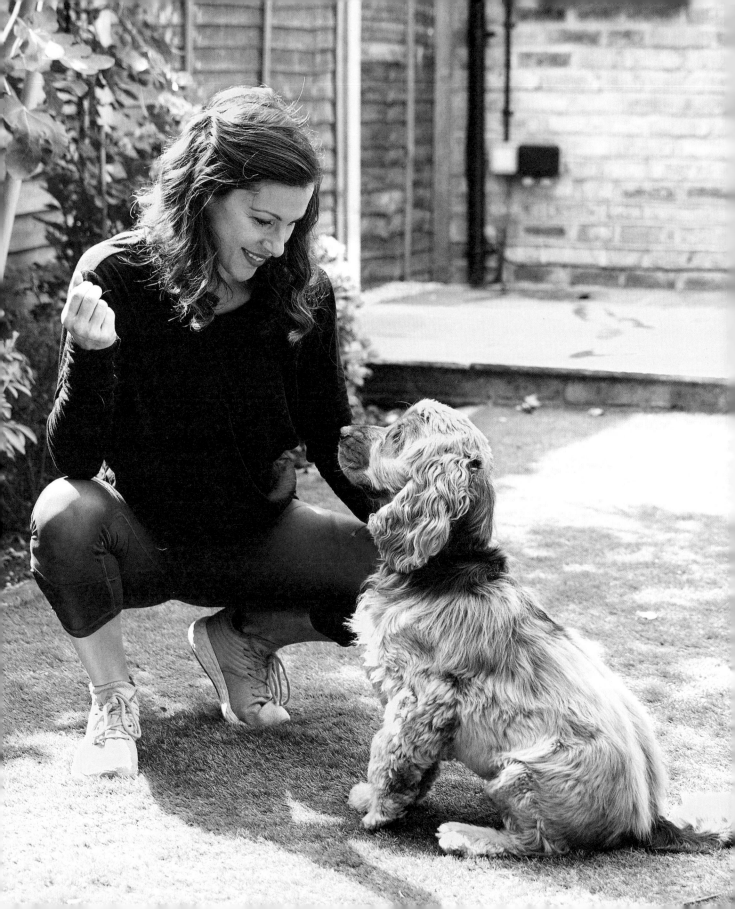

FIRST TRIMESTER

1-12 WEEKS

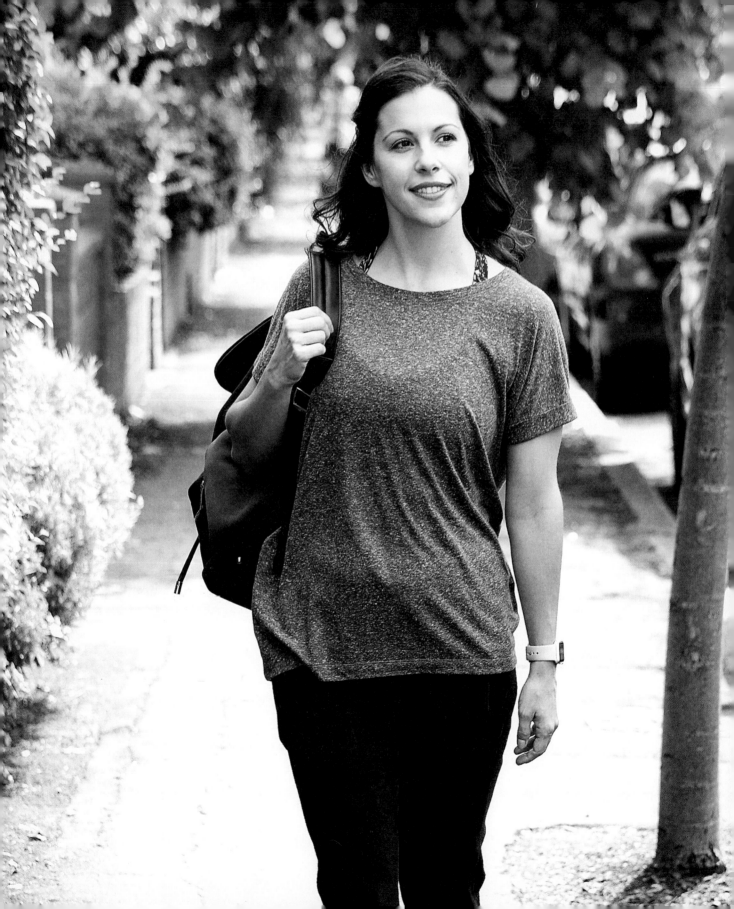

Great Expectations

You're expecting! Isn't this a funny way to describe pregnancy? Yes it's so full of expectation – excitement over meeting your baby in nine months' time, anxiety about what those nine months will bring, a fierce and sudden maternal instinct to prevent any harm coming to the life inside you. Yet, at the same time, almost every aspect of pregnancy will surprise you. If you're one for comparing yourself to others, or even to yourself, it's time to let those expectations go.

No two pregnancies will be the same – even a subsequent pregnancy, if this is not your first nine-month victory march. However, there are a number of physiological changes you *can* expect to take place, and the first trimester packs in plenty of them.

Let's talk about the weeks of pregnancy. Most expecting mums only discover they're pregnant after their first missed period – I was rather flustered to learn that six weeks had flown by without me realising! Some women remain unaware of their pregnancy for eight or even twelve weeks, by which time any first-trimester symptoms should be signposting some less than ordinary activity.

We'll discuss your baby's development each month but, rest assured, as abstract as that life within may feel, in these few short months your baby will become a fully fledged mini human with a beating heart, all its other vital organs and even little finger- and toenails. That means your body has a lot of work to do. So, whether you're early in your pregnancy journey or catching up on what's been going on beneath the bump, here's what the first trimester means for you.

Your Changing Body

Yogis have coined a phrase that I feel perfectly summarises your first trimester health outlook: working *in*. Whether the circumstances of your first trimester allow you to work out almost daily or during infrequent nausea-free moments, there is a head-to-toe 24/7 workout underway within your body. Arm yourself with knowledge, turn up your intuition and remember to work *in* to get more from your work*outs*.

BRAIN

It's completely normal to feel tired, emotional or anxious, and to struggle to focus in the first trimester – a sharp influx of hormones means your brain is receiving and transmitting more signals than ever. Exercise aids endorphin release, helping to promote a better hormonal balance and a more stable mood.

STOMACH

It's unknown why some women experience morning sickness and others don't, but the cocktail of hormones required to create a healthy home for your baby can certainly make you feel off-centre. Drinking ample water, eating small frequent snacks and low-key aerobic exercise can help offset nausea, which should ease by the second trimester.

HEART

Your blood vessels expand almost immediately when you become pregnant, so your heart has to pump faster in order to keep up with circulatory demands. If you wear a fitness tracker, training at around eighty per cent of your maximum heart rate should prevent overexertion.

BREASTS

Your breasts are the first place you'll feel the effect of increased oestrogen and progesterone production in the womb. You'll begin to store extra fat here and they will probably feel more sensitive. Size up in your favourite supportive bras to avoid discomfort from impact.

OVARIES

The ovaries produce progesterone, which creates a safe uterine environment for baby, and oestrogen, which helps to regulate production of other essential pregnancy hormones, such as relaxin. Relaxin reaches its highest level in the first trimester, working to soften the blood vessels, muscle tissues and ligaments to meet the new demands of pregnancy. For this reason, the first trimester workouts will teach you how to strengthen and stabilise your joints.

PLACENTA

Human chorionic gonadotropin (hCG) is produced by the placenta and communicates with the ovaries to regulate hormone production throughout pregnancy. For the first six weeks, hCG levels can double every two days – a development that is often cited as the cause for morning sickness. It's these high levels of hCG that allow us to detect pregnancy as early as three days after implantation.

BLADDER

Your uterus is already expanding to make space for the developing embryo. Until your stomach stretches to accommodate the growth, there is going to be some extra pressure on your bladder. Use the additional toilet breaks to move around and boost circulation.

BLOOD VESSELS

Blood volume will rise gradually throughout pregnancy, culminating in a fifty per cent increase by week 34. Before it does, the blood vessels will dilate in preparation. Early in this transition - particularly in the first trimester - you may experience some light-headedness due to temporary 'vascular underfill' (resulting in low blood pressure). Try to avoid sudden position changes that may throw you off balance.

Power to Your Pelvic Floor

A hammock-like network of muscles, ligaments and connective tissue lining the base of your pelvis, the pelvic floor has two key functions: the first is to support your digestive and reproductive organs; the second is to promote engagement of the deep-core muscles, which support and guide the spine during exercise and everyday active living.

The average woman holds at least 11.5kg (25lb) of extra weight by the end of her pregnancy, which means that her pelvic floor has to work extra hard to support the organs. Daily pelvic floor exercises throughout pregnancy help to strengthen this vital network of muscles and can decrease incontinence in the third trimester as well as during the postpartum period. It's far easier to prevent disorders of the pelvic floor than it is to rehabilitate them, so it's worth starting early.

BASIC PELVIC FLOOR EXERCISES
Perform these simple exercises three to four times a day.

- Without clenching your glutes or stomach muscles, subtly lift your pelvic floor from the back passage towards the front. Think of the muscle gently rolling as you squeeze. Practise holding for up to ten seconds in one contraction, then reset and repeat for a total of ten reps. These will promote endurance of the pelvic floor muscles through slow-twitch muscle fibres.

- Practise faster squeezes too. Squeeze and hold for just one second, rest for one second, and repeat for ten reps. This will promote rapid engagement of the fast-twitch muscle fibres when you sneeze, cough or jump.

GET MORE FROM YOUR PELVIC FLOOR TRAINING

Daily squeezing will strengthen the pelvic floor, but you can get even more from proper activation of this muscle group by training it in a way that's relevant to everyday movements. Here's how:

REPOSITION REGULARLY Start practising your pelvic floor squeezes by lying down, as it's easier to detect if you're squeezing the bigger surrounding muscles instead. If the glutes press into the floor, make the movement smaller and more isolated.

Once you've mastered lying squeezes, alternate your position every set so you can activate the muscles during a variety of everyday movements. Try to do one set daily in each of the following positions: lying, seated, on all fours and standing.

BLOW BEFORE YOU GO Pair your squeezes with your breath. Use the phrase 'blow before you go' to remind you to exhale as you engage your pelvic floor. Think about simultaneously breathing down and lifting the muscles up. This is also the proper way to lift weights (or a suitcase, for that matter). As you inhale, breathe in and up into your diaphragm and simultaneously relax your pelvic floor down.

BUCKLE UP Use your pelvic floor to trigger subtle engagement of your transverse abdominis muscle. Think of these deep-lying core muscles as a belt buckle that you're clicking together. Slowly roll the pelvic floor forwards, then gently tighten beneath your belly button. If you hold your hands around your waist, you shouldn't feel your obliques contract. Learning this subtle muscle connection now can help guard against abdominal separation.

MOVE MINDFULLY Once you've mastered the above training methods, use your breath and pelvic floor engagement while you move. For instance, as you lower into a squat you will inhale and relax your pelvic floor. As you stand you will exhale and engage your pelvic floor. Remember always to exhale on the exertion. For more repetitive activities such as running, try relaxing the muscles for a count of four as you inhale, and contracting the muscles for a count of four as you exhale.

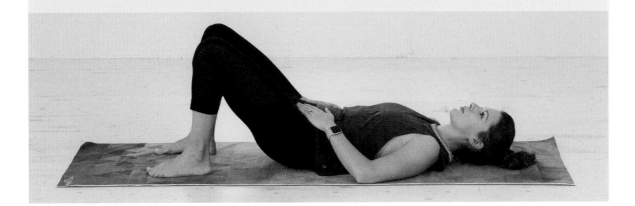

Beginnings & Endings

During pregnancy, the onslaught of physical changes can feel like a strange out-of-body experience. Bookending your workouts with the following warm-up and cool-down will help you reassume residence in your body, safely increase and decrease your respiratory rate and body temperature, clock any changes to your range of motion, and establish a more mindful awareness of the muscles that play a starring role during your unique nine-month production.

FIRST TRIMESTER WARM-UP

Perform each of these five exercises for one set, paying particular attention to the relationship between your breathing and the contraction of your pelvic floor and transverse abdominis (see pages 28-29). The earlier you engage the pelvic floor correctly during workouts, the more resilient your body will be to the abdominal stretching and pelvic floor stress that comes later in pregnancy.

SLOW SWAN DIVES

1. Stand in a neutral position with your feet hip-width apart. From here, inhale while you sweep your arms overhead and stretch through your spine.
2. As you exhale, fold forward from your hips and bring your hands down to your shins or knees, allowing your shoulders to round gently.
3. Inhale and pull your shoulder blades together so that your back flattens. Exhale as you rise back to standing. That's one rep.

CAT COWS

1. Come to all fours with your shoulders over your hands and your hips over your knees. As you exhale, round your spine away from the floor and scoop your navel in. Practise gently lifting your pelvic floor as you do so.
2. As you inhale, soften your belly towards the floor and look up to the sky. Pause to feel the stretch across your shoulders and lumbar, relaxing your pelvic floor in preparation for the next rep.

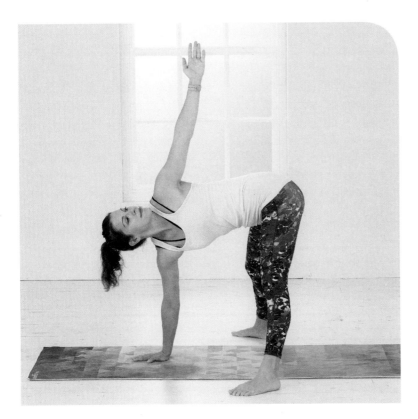

WIDE-LEG TORSO TWISTS

1. In a neutral position, stand with your feet in a wide stance and come to your flat back folded position, hands either on your knees or on the floor if your hamstrings are flexible.
2. Keep one hand planted as you roll the opposite arm towards the sky. Resist rotating your hip as you stretch through your chest and shoulders.
3. Both sides make up one rep. Practise breathing out to open the arm, and breathing in to return to centre.

PLANK STEPS

1. Tuck your toes and come into a high plank position. Make sure your elbows stay soft and your quads remain lifted so that your lower back is flat, not dipped.
2. Step your right foot 45 degrees to the side, without rotating or dropping the hips. Return to centre and repeat on the other side. That's one rep.

DEEP SQUATS

1. Stand with your feet hip-width apart and toes slightly turned out. Drop your bum as low as you can without your chest rounding or heels lifting.
2. Make sure your knees track over your toes throughout the movement – they will want to roll in, so gently drive them out to the sides.
3. At the bottom of the move, check that you can lift your toes. If you've rolled onto the balls of your feet, you've gone deeper than your flexibility allows. Always work within the range that's safe and comfortable for your body. Inhale as you lower and exhale as you stand.

FIRST TRIMESTER COOL-DOWN

Work through each of these stretches to reset your heart rate and body temperature gradually. Pregnancy hormones can cause both to become more irregular in the first trimester. The stretches shine a spotlight on the muscles that become tightest as your body changes; optimise their mobility now and you'll thank yourself later, when you successfully steer clear of muscular imbalances and back pain.

KNEELING CHEST STRETCH

1. Adopt a high kneeling position and place your hands on your lower back. Gently engage your glutes and drive your hips forward as you draw your elbows together.
2. If you feel strong and stable in your back, you could bring one hand to the heel of the foot on the same side and open the other hand to the sky. Make sure your glutes remain engaged if you do so.
3. Hold the stretch for ten to fifteen seconds.

WALKING CHILD'S POSE

1. From kneeling, allow your hips to melt back over your heels, your chest to fall gently over your thighs and your hands to stretch out in front of you. If you feel bloated in this position, try taking your knees wider than your hips.
2. Keeping your hips stable, laterally walk your hands over to one side until you feel a stretch down the opposite side of your body. Pause for a few breaths before walking to the other side.

TWISTED RUNNER

1. From a high plank, bring your right foot outside your right hand and allow your left knee to drop to the mat behind you. Using your right hand, gently push the right knee out to the side and twist your chest towards the knee.
2. You should feel the release in your middle back and outer hip. Enjoy a few deep breaths here before switching sides.

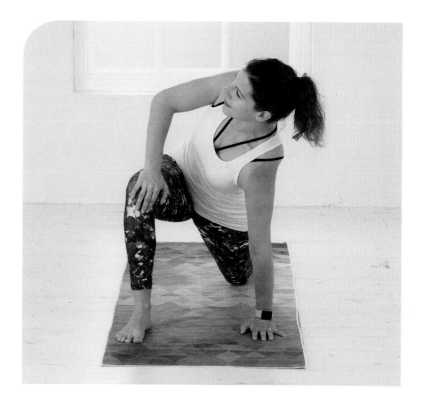

FINDING NEUTRAL POSITION

Your first trimester is the best time to get comfortable in neutral position, as it becomes increasingly difficult to find as your pregnancy progresses. Here's how to find it:

1. Lie on your back with your knees bent and heels 30cm (12in) away from your bum.
2. Rock your hips gently forwards and drive your navel down so your lower back presses firmly into the floor.
3. Now drive your pelvis back and allow your lower back to form a gentle arch from your bum to your shoulders.
4. Rock three to four times between these two positions, then settle at the midpoint where you can comfortably contract your rib cage while maintaining a sliver of daylight under your lower back.
5. This is your neutral position. Repeat steps three and four of this exercise on your feet, using a wall if you find the pressure against your bum and shoulders a helpful point of reference.

PIGEON

1. From an all-fours position, bring your right shin forward across your body, so your right heel rests in front of your left hip. Allow your left thigh to soften to the floor behind you.
2. Simultaneously soften into both hips, encouraging your right hip towards the floor and your left hip towards your right foot.
3. Keep this movement static and enjoy a few deep breaths, or make it dynamic and alternate between rounding and opening your shoulders to massage your middle back. Repeat on the other side.

SIDE BODY

1. Find a comfortable cross-legged position and plant your right palm 30cm (12in) away from your right hip.
2. Without lifting your left hip, reach your left arm overhead and towards the right. You should feel the stretch along the side of your body.
3. Lengthen on the inhale and reach a little further on the exhale until you can feel the stretch in your diaphragm and obliques. Repeat on the other side.

HAMSTRING STRETCH

1. From your seated position, extend one leg in front of you and pull your toes back towards you.
2. If you don't feel the stretch in your hamstring, sit tall through your spine and fold gently over the leg. Hold the deepest position for a few breaths, then switch sides.

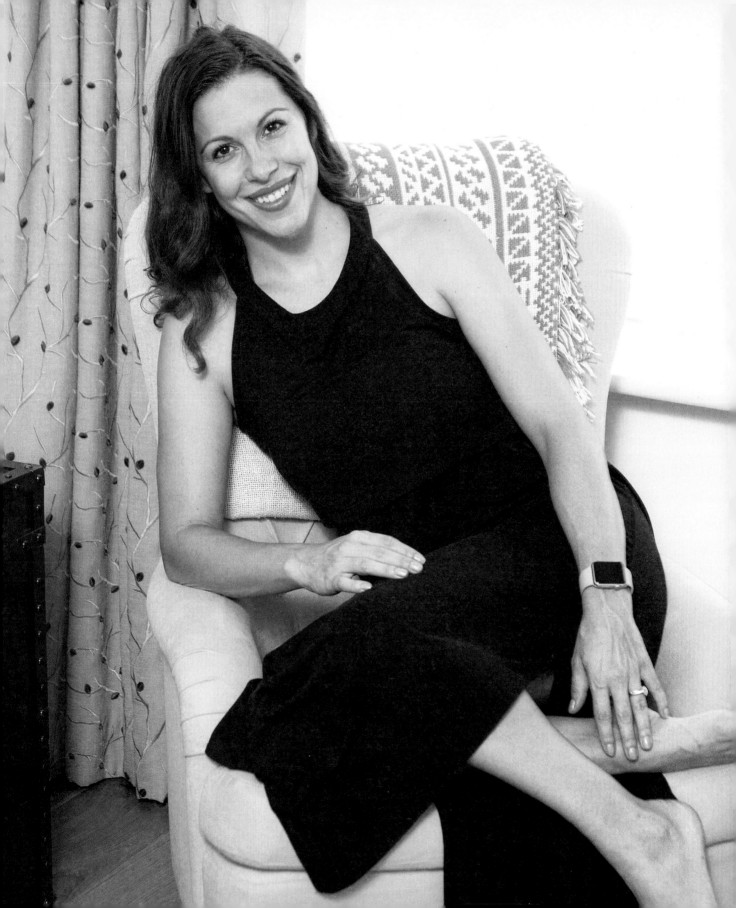

Month One Wellness Agenda

As it's not always possible to detect pregnancy just yet, you may be using this month's workouts while trying for a baby or as an introductory few weeks of training before moving onto the month two workouts. Wherever you are in your conception or early pregnancy journey, your primary goal now is to lay down the foundations for a strong and active pregnancy.

- Channel any nerves about conception or pregnancy into a constructive outlet and reap the emotional benefits of regular endorphin release.

- Rehearse the major movement patterns you'll be mastering during the *MBB* nine-month programme.

- Strengthen the muscles and joints that will be fundamental to a strong, injury-free pregnancy. They are:

  - *Transverse abdominis* to support posture and prevent abdominal separation.

  - *Obliques* to aid deep-core engagement and prevent injury during rotational movement.

  - *Erector spinae* and *quadratus lumborum* to support the lower back and reduce postural change and back pain.

  - *Gluteus muscles (glutes)* and *hamstrings* to prevent over-lengthening and weakening against the pull of your bump.

  - Muscles of the upper back – notably the *latissimus dorsi (lats)*, *rear deltoids (delts)* and *rhomboids* – to aid upright posture against the pull of heavier breasts and in preparation for the repetitive rounding of shoulders while baby-soothing and breastfeeding.

  - *All major joints* to counteract an increase of relaxin and to optimise stability for strength training and everyday movement.

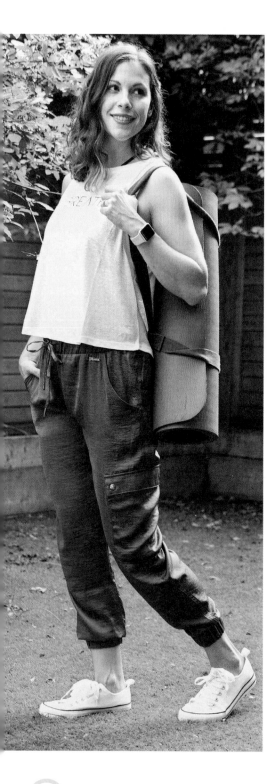

What is Happening to Your Body?

WHAT?

Most women learn they're pregnant after month one, as many symptoms are subtle before this time. Very early signs of pregnancy include fatigue, bloating and sore breasts. If your periods run like clockwork, an unusual delay in week five may well be the first indication. As the embryo implants, it can sometimes shed a little of the uterine lining. In some cases this light bleeding is enough to postpone the revelatory moment for yet another month.

WHY?

Although month one includes weeks one to four of your pregnancy, you're technically only pregnant from around week two, when the egg is fertilised. It takes roughly one more week to implant and for the placenta to form, beginning production of the primary pregnancy hormone hCG and, with it, an increase in oestrogen, progesterone and relaxin. This sudden surge of hormones is the reason why your pregnancy test comes up positive.

SO WHAT?

You may experience mixed emotions when you first discover you're pregnant, so give yourself time to absorb and celebrate the news. If you've been trying for a baby and are reading this book in preparation for a fit pregnancy, you may already be doing the month one workouts. You'll probably still feel like your pre-pregnancy self, so make a strong start on your prenatal training now and it will be easier to stick to when month two symptoms kick in.

What is Happening to Your Baby?

BENEATH THE BUMP

While its home is in the early stages of 'bump construction', your baby has plenty to report in month one. Once the egg is fertilised around week two, it becomes an embryo and grows into a mass of cells (a blastocyst), which makes up the foundations of fetal development. Around the three-week mark, that blastocyst will implant in your uterus.

Growing to the size of a poppy seed, the blastocyst will organise itself into three layers that make up the foundations for the baby's brain, skeleton and muscle, and respiratory and digestive organs. In order to aid this development and nourish your baby, a placenta is beginning to develop and will become fully functional at around ten weeks. In the meantime, baby is getting all its nourishment from a protective fluid-filled amniotic sac.

BUILDING AN ATHLETE

The next nine months present a uniquely empowering process during which you can play a very active role in your baby's development. The most important thing you can do in the very early weeks (and even before falling pregnant) is take a folic acid supplement to support fetal development. These early stages of pregnancy are when adequate intake of this very special B vitamin matters most, as it helps the neural tube develop into a healthy brain and spinal cord.

Although some foods are fortified with folic acid, it can be difficult to get sufficient quantities through food alone, so midwives recommend supplementing 400mcg daily until you are twelve weeks pregnant. Most prenatal multivitamins will include folic acid, so check the label to give your baby the best possible start.

BABY PBs

Only fifty per cent of fertilised eggs survive until implantation, so your fledgling baby is already performing above average.

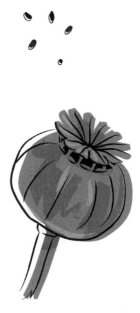

Energy-Boost Countdown

When you first learn you're pregnant, you may find those first few weeks wildly exciting or quietly anxious – know that both reactions are completely natural. When your little secret is stirring big emotions, this countdown-style workout will keep your mind centred and your body strong with endorphin-boosting pregnancy-safe movements.

Use the first trimester warm-up (page 30) to prepare your body and mind ahead of this equipment-free workout. Complete ten reps of each exercise, transitioning to the next move as quickly as possible until you complete the final exercise. Rest when you need to, being mindful to stay hydrated and to respect your body if you feel low in energy. Enjoy a longer rest of up to two minutes after each full round. Return to the first exercise and complete eight reps of each exercise throughout. Continue dropping by two reps per round until your fifth and final round takes you to two reps of each exercise. Catch your breath with the cool-down (page 32).

Mindful Mamas
Look out for modifications and aim to complete the countdown in under thirty minutes.

Tandem Athletes
Move as quickly and energetically as you can while maintaining good form. Aim to complete the countdown in under twenty-five minutes.

MOUNTAIN CLIMBERS

1. Assume a high plank position with a gentle bend in your elbows, your shoulders rolling away from the ground and your quads engaged. A strong plank should look a little rounded across the back of your body, with a slight hollowing under your abdomen.

2. Maintain tension and stability in your upper body as you drive one knee to your chest at a time. Two knees make up one rep.

Modification: Keep one foot on the ground at a time rather than switching in midair.

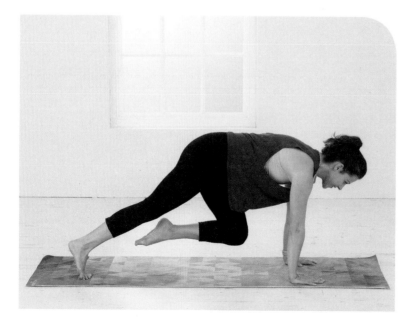

ALTERNATING REVERSE LUNGE KICK

1. Stand with your feet hip-width apart and your pelvis tucked under your rib cage.
2. Drive your right leg back and bend both knees to ninety degrees, making sure the left knee tracks over the toe.
3. Brace your core and push through your left foot as you sweep your right leg beneath and in front of you into a high kick.
4. Return to standing and repeat on the other leg. That's one rep.

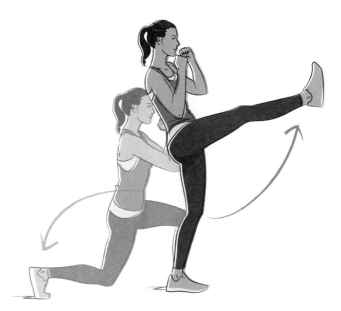

ALTERNATING SIDE LUNGES

1. Stand with your feet hip-width apart and your pelvis tucked under your rib cage.
2. Drive your right foot out to the side and transfer your weight into your right hip as you drop your bum in line with your knee.
3. Check your feet are still parallel at the bottom of the lunge and your knee is pointing forward.
4. Brace your core and push off your right foot to return to standing. Repeat on the left. That's one rep.

Modification: If you find it challenging to keep the feet parallel after each step, simply hold a wide-leg stance while shifting your weight from one side to the other.

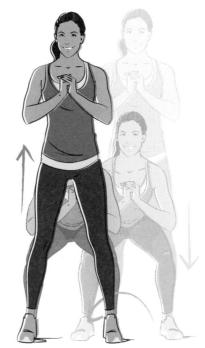

SHUFFLE SQUAT

1. Keep your feet hip-width apart and your weight in your heels throughout this exercise.
2. Drop your hips into a deep squat, keeping your knees over your ankles and your chest upright.
3. Take a wide step or 'shuffle' with both feet, then squeeze your glutes to stand.
4. Alternate direction every rep.

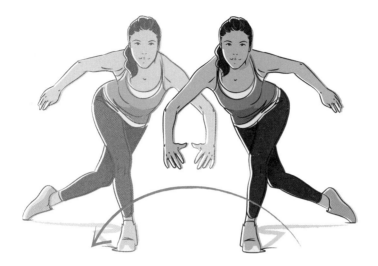

SKATER JUMPS

1. From standing, push off your left foot to move energetically to the right. Land with a soft bend in your right knee and continue lowering your hips to touch your left hand gently to your right ankle.
2. As you lift up, push off your right foot and over to the left side. That's one rep.

Modification: Try stepping energetically from side to side instead of jumping.

INCLINE TRICEP PRESS-UPS

1. Use an elevated platform – a bench, chair or sofa – and assume an incline plank position with soft elbows, slightly rounded shoulders and engaged quads.
2. With your hands directly under your shoulders and your elbows pointing straight back, lower your chest. Exhale to return.
3. Keep your back slightly rounded and core subtly hollowed to support your lumbar spine.

Modification: If your elbows flare out or you feel any pressure in your lower back, do this on your knees with your hips tucked in line with your rib cage.

TRICEP DIPS

1. Using the same platform, face the other way and support yourself on your hands, fingers facing forward and elbows pointing straight back.
2. Lower your body until your elbows are ninety degrees, keeping your spine as upright as possible.
3. Increase or decrease the challenge by stepping your feet further away or bringing them closer.

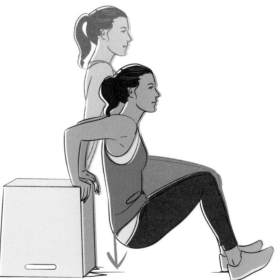

PLANK CROSS-BODY TOE TAPS

1. Assume a high plank position, repeating all your form checks – soft elbows, rounded shoulders, quads engaged.
2. Transfer your weight into your left hand as you energetically drive your hips into a deep upside-down V and bring your right hand across to your left ankle.
3. Return to your plank and repeat on the other side. That's one rep.

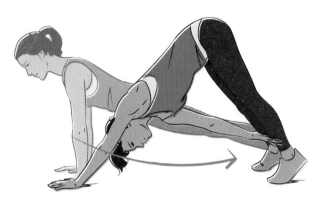

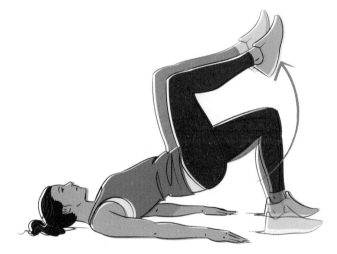

MARCHING BRIDGE HOLD

1. Lie on your back with your feet close together, knees bent and stacked over your ankles.
2. Roll through your spine to lift your hips until there's a straight line from your collarbone to your knees.
3. Hold this position – glutes engaged and hips level – as you lift one shin parallel to the floor. Hold for a second before repeating on the other side. That's one rep.

Modification: If you are doing this workout after month five, rest your mid-back on an elevated platform like a sofa, Swiss ball or bench so your heart remains above or level with your hips.

SIDE PLANK HIP DROPS

1. Assume a side plank on your elbows, anchoring between either your elbow and your knees or your elbow and the sides of your feet.
2. Soften your shoulder away from your ear to make sure you're doing the work in your obliques rather than in your back or shoulders.
3. Allow your hip to drop softly towards the floor, then lift it away from the floor until there's a slight rainbow shape along your midline.
4. Do all your reps on one side before switching over.

Strong Mum Foundations

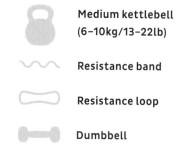

45 mins

Use your first resistance workout to rehearse the major movement patterns you'll be revisiting and revising over the months to come. Already you will start to strengthen the muscles down the back of your body to prepare them for the anterior pull effect that your bump will eventually create. Unilateral movements, which emphasise one side of the body at a time, will also help to strengthen your joints – the *MBB* antidote to a sharp rise in the ligament-softening hormone relaxin.

Fully mobilise your body with the warm-up (page 30) before tackling the Strong Mum Foundations workout. Make your weight and rep choice according to the Mindful Mama or Tandem Athlete guidelines. Complete three rounds of circuits one and two, working through each exercise consecutively. For the stability superset, complete a total of six rounds; alternate the working side each round, or, for an added challenge, complete three consecutive rounds on one side then three rounds on the other. Remember to lengthen the muscles you've strengthened with the cool-down (page 32).

Mindful Mamas

For circuit one, choose a light weight that allows you to complete fifteen reps of each exercise. Do ten reps of each exercise in circuit two and the stability superset.

Tandem Athletes

For circuit one, choose a heavier weight that allows you to complete ten reps of each exercise. Do twelve to fifteen reps of each exercise in circuit two and the stability superset.

CIRCUIT ONE

SUMO DEADLIFT

1. Stand with your feet just over hip-width apart, toes turned out slightly. Softly bend your knees to pick up the kettlebell from between your feet, hinging from the hips and maintaining a flat back as you stand.
2. Push your hips into the kettlebell at the top of the movement. You should feel the work in your hamstrings and your bum, but you should never feel any pain in your lower back.
3. Return the kettlebell to your mid-shin and repeat. Be sure that you're 'pulling' through the back body and not pushing through the front of your thighs.

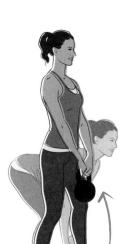

Equipment

Medium kettlebell (6–10kg/13–22lb)

Resistance band

Resistance loop

Dumbbell

GOBLET SUMO SQUAT

1. Hold a kettlebell upside down, squeezing it firmly in front of your chest. Maintain the same turned-out sumo position with your feet and ensure your knees track over your toes as you lower down.
2. At the base of your squat, check that you can lift your toes towards the sky. Draw your inner thighs together and squeeze the glutes to stand.
3. Move smoothly and without momentum, ensuring there is no bounce at the bottom of your squat and no jolting into the knees at the top.

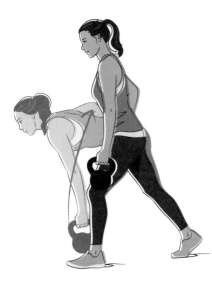

SPLIT-STANCE DEADLIFT

1. Adopt a split stance with one foot 30–60cm (1–2ft) in front of the other. Keep the knees soft.
2. Holding a kettlebell outside your front thigh, send your hips back and fold with a flat back until the kettlebell reaches your mid-shin. Use your front hamstring and glute to pull yourself back to standing, realigning your pelvis under your rib cage at the top.
3. Keep the hip of your back leg stable and pointing forward throughout. This is a more stable variation of a single-leg deadlift, making it a great choice for strengthening your posterior body during pregnancy.

CIRCUIT TWO

PLANK ROW

1. In a high plank position, wrap both your thumbs around a resistance loop. Keep your shoulders over your hands and a gentle bend in your elbows.
2. Shifting your weight into one palm, pull the other hand into your waist. Your elbow should point directly behind you.
3. Keep hugging your belly button away from the earth and lifting your quads. This will strengthen your stomach and back at once.

Modification: Lower the knees into a three-quarter plank position if you require more lumbar support or pelvic stability.

RECLINE HIGH ROWS

1. In a seated position with your knees gently bent in front of you, wrap a resistance band around your heels and create a soft C curve with your spine as you lower your shoulders roughly forty-five degrees to the floor.
2. Holding both ends of the resistance band, keep your navel scooped into your spine and draw one elbow high and in line with your shoulder, gently twisting the shoulder in the same direction. Repeat to the other side. That's one rep.
3. Resist being too straight in your back, which could put pressure on your lumbar, or too relaxed in the shoulders. Although your back is gently curved, deeply hug your spine with the core muscles either side of it. This way you will strengthen your stomach and back muscles simultaneously.

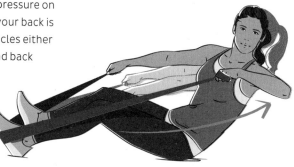

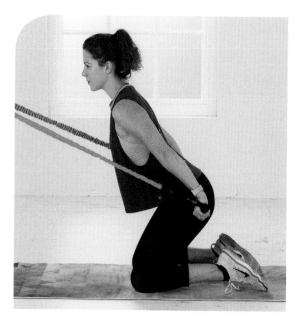

KNEELING SHOULDER OPENERS

1. Wrap a long resistance band around a pole, tree or banister (anything sturdy that won't topple over as you pull against it). Come to a high kneeling position with tension in the band as you hold either side of it about 30cm (12in) in front of you.
2. Draw your navel in and, without moving your torso, exhale and pull the ends of the band to the sides of your hips. Inhale and return, maintaining control against resistance.
3. You should feel this in your lats and core, plus you'll strengthen the stabilising ligaments of your hips and shoulders in the process.

STABILITY SUPERSET

Instructions specify one side for clarity. Switch the dominant arm and leg each round or after all three rounds, as per your chosen intensity level.

ALL-FOURS FLY

1. With a light dumbbell in your right hand, come to an all-fours position and gently scoop your tailbone to engage your core.
2. Transfer your weight into your left hand and exhale to raise your weighted hand out to the side in line with your shoulder, without twisting through your hips. Inhale back to centre.

Modification: If this is very easy, try lifting and lowering the left leg simultaneously with the opposite arm.

BURPEE TO LUNGE PRESS

1. Keeping the dumbbell in the right hand, come to a high plank position. Jump your feet softly forwards and push through your heels to stand.
2. Once standing, drop the right leg back into a deep lunge while pushing the right arm towards the sky.
3. Step back through centre, lower the weight and plant the hands to jump back to a high plank.

Modification: Step rather than jump if you feel less energetic or require less impact. Elevate your hands on a bench if you feel light-headed during sudden position changes.

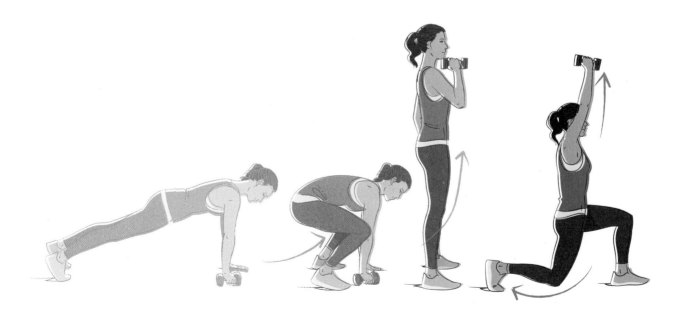

Month Two Wellness Agenda

If you are going to get morning sickness, it usually rears its nauseating head by month two. You may not feel like moving much, but turning your focus onto something positive can help to reduce feelings of restlessness and lethargy.

- Use movement as a healthy outlet for anxiety and a distraction from morning sickness; maintain a level of exertion that reduces your symptoms and always stop if you begin to feel worse.

- When performing back-to-back exercises, select movements that are on the same plane to reduce blood flow demand and feelings of faintness. For example, pair standing exercises together rather than changing suddenly from standing to sitting or lying.

- Simplify your workouts to include fewer exercises, helping you stay focused and present while you train.

- Continue prioritising muscles that will help you feel more centred and stable, including the core and the glutes.

BERRY BREAKFAST SMOOTHIE

Serves One

100g (3½oz) frozen banana
30g (1oz) frozen blueberries
30g (1oz) frozen raspberries
½ tsp ground cinnamon
20g (¾oz) oats
1 tbsp peanut butter
Milk of choice

350 calories · 62g carbs · 8g protein · 9g fat (excluding milk)

Low blood sugar and poor hydration are two of the biggest triggers of morning sickness. If you can't stomach anything more solid in the mornings, try this delicious smoothie and hydrate as you nourish. The fats in the peanut butter will slow the absorption of fructose from the fruit, while cinnamon is known to reduce insulin sensitivity to stabilise blood sugar.

To make, blitz all the ingredients in a blender. Pour into a glass and enjoy.

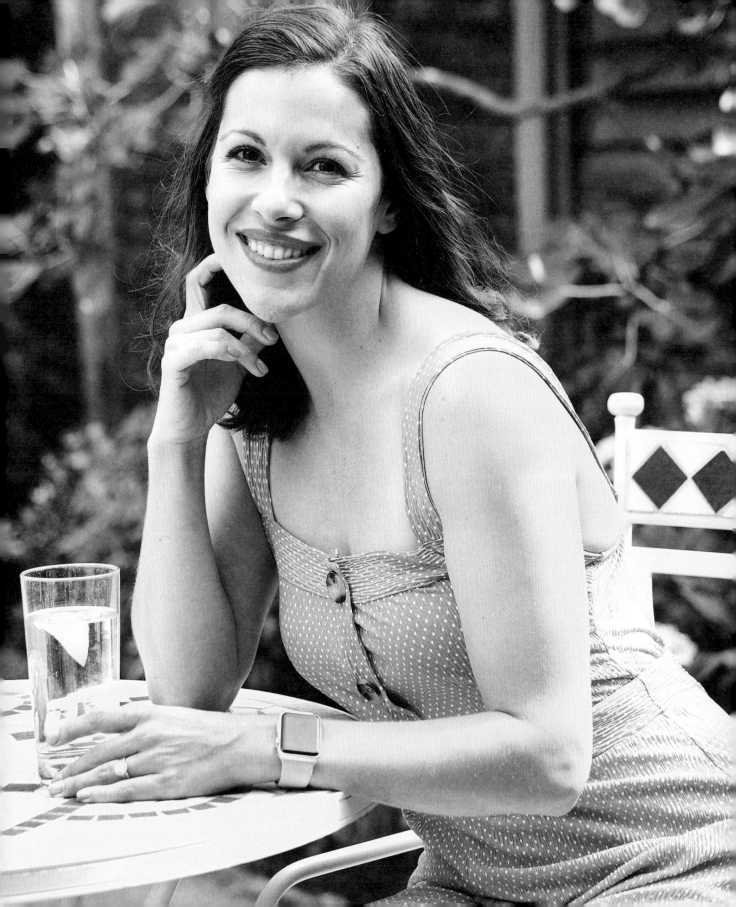

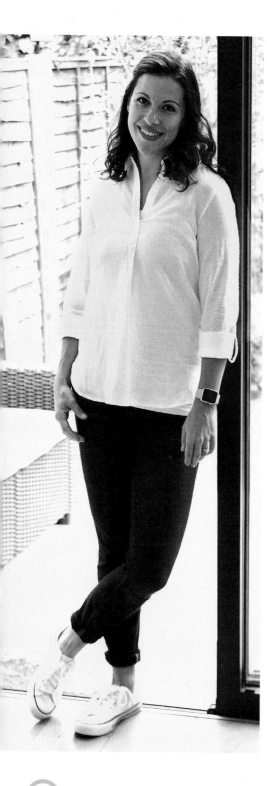

What is Happening to Your Body?

WHAT?

This month is when most mums-to-be have their revelatory moment. If a missed period doesn't do it, the nausea and fatigue we associate with morning sickness will almost certainly tip you off. Everyone has a unique experience of their first trimester, so don't be hard on yourself if you're feeling particularly drained. Likewise, don't be alarmed if your symptoms are few and far between – we all respond differently to the physiological changes taking place.

WHY?

The post-implantation hormone hCG is on the rise, and rapidly. It will almost double every two to three days as the placenta develops, causing much of the nausea and fatigue we associate with morning sickness. The placenta requires nourishment from nutrients in your blood supply, so your blood vessels will now dilate in preparation for increased blood volume. This process takes time, so you may feel a little faint as your blood pressure initially drops off and your heart rate increases to compensate for the change.

SO WHAT?

Dehydration can make other symptoms worse, especially if you're vomiting, so take on plenty of water. If you feel dizzy, avoid weight training and opt instead for walks in the fresh air. Nausea feels invariably worse when you're sedentary, so the endorphin release of light exercise will provide a welcome distraction when you can manage it. If you do try some strength training, avoid raising your arms overhead or making sudden position changes, as this will increase faintness while your blood pressure is lowered.

What is Happening to Your Baby?

BENEATH THE BUMP

Your little poppy seed will grow to the size of a raspberry this month, and as baby makes the transition from embryo to fetus by week eight, two key organs are taking shape.

The heart is one of the first organs to develop, and by week six a heartbeat is usually detectable by ultrasound. As baby's little body begins to circulate blood, a string of vessels also connects him or her to your placenta. This will become the umbilical cord and will provide all baby's nourishment once the placenta is advanced enough to take on the job.

The neural tube that formed in month one also develops rapidly into the brain and spinal cord. In fact, brain growth is so rapid that baby's head visibly expands and becomes disproportionate to the rest of its body. Limb buds will appear as a forerunner to arms and legs (and soon to fingers and toes), so the rest of your fledgling will follow suit shortly.

BUILDING AN ATHLETE

If your pregnancy was unexpected, you may not have been taking folic acid supplements. Now is the time to start, as baby's neural development is underway and this will help to ensure a healthy brain and spine. Speaking of your brainy baby, research shows that even twenty minutes of heart-rate-elevating exercise (a brisk walk counts) three times a week from early pregnancy increases brain activity in newborns, so rest assured your little prodigy is already benefitting from your proactive start to an active pregnancy!

BABY PBs

By the end of this month, baby looks a lot more baby-like. A fully fledged fetus at eight weeks, its primary organs are now developed and all that remains is more growth to prepare for life on the outside.

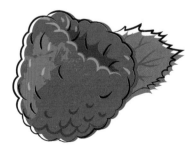

The Body Balancer

This simple bodyweight workout introduces some more advanced core-strengthening movements. You'll play with unilateral balance exercises that require mindful integration of the breath. This in turn activates the autonomic nervous system, reducing the stress response that often exaggerates those feelings of nausea.

After your warm-up (page 30), set a stopwatch and get ready to move **e**very **m**inute, **o**n the **m**inute (it's EMOM time). Start with ten reps of the squat crunch then perform the squat hold until one minute finishes and the next begins. Repeat this for ten rounds. Next complete circuit two for two or three rounds, according to your chosen level, followed by circuit three. You should build a nice heat in the legs, which you'll gently release with the cool-down (page 32).

Mindful Mamas

For circuits one and two, complete two rounds of ten reps. In circuit two, do all the exercises on one leg, then swap sides. That's one round.

Tandem Athletes

For circuits one and two, complete three rounds of twelve reps. In circuit two, do all the exercises on one leg for three rounds, then complete three rounds on the other side.

EMOM SUPERSET

SQUAT CRUNCH

1. With your toes in a slight turnout and your arms bent in line with your shoulders, palms facing forwards, perform a basic squat.
2. As you rise from your squat, transfer your weight into one foot and squeeze the opposite knee out and up towards your elbow. Make sure you're squeezing knee to elbow and not elbow to knee.
3. Repeat on the other side. That's one rep. This one should be fast but controlled – no bouncing at the bottom or jolting at the top.

Equipment

Set of double-sided gliders

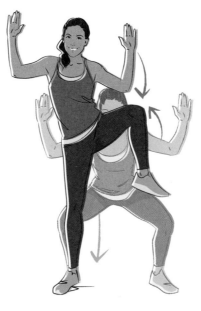

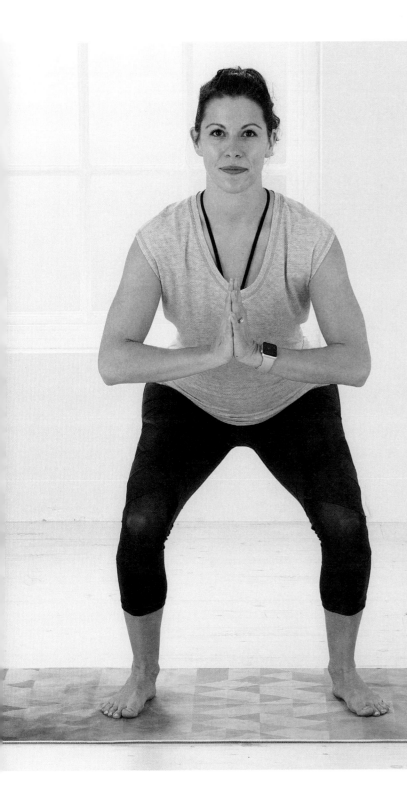

SQUAT HOLD

1. Drop to the lowest point of your squat, where you can safely distribute most of your weight in the heels and keep your chest pointing forwards.

2. Hold this position, making sure the knees track over the toes. Catch your breath, engaging the pelvic floor with every exhale and relaxing the pelvic floor with every inhale.

CIRCUIT ONE

BRIDGE CURLS

1. Lie on your back with your knees bent and both heels resting on gliders. Peel your lower back off the floor until there's a straight line between your collarbone and your hip bones.
2. Without rolling your hips, extend one leg away.
3. Return to centre and extend the other leg away. That's one rep.

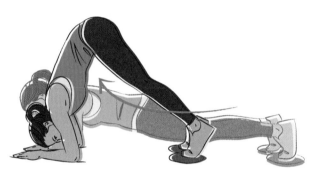

FOREARM PIKE

1. Assume a low plank position with your toes resting on gliders.
2. Initiating the movement from your belly button, slowly pull the gliders towards your elbows and send your hips to the sky.
3. Actively relaxing the top of your shoulders away from your ears and lengthening under your armpits will ensure that the work comes from your core and not from your shoulders.

ROLLING PRESS-UP

1. A great advanced move that, together with good breathing technique, will help you prevent abdominal separation in later pregnancy. In a three-quarter plank position, with a straight line from the back of your neck to the back of your knees, and with your hands on gliders, slowly roll one glider forward while lowering into a press-up with the opposite arm.
2. Inhale to roll out and press down; exhale to return to centre. Imagine there's a piece of string running down your back – it shouldn't dip or peak around your lower back if you're maintaining constant gentle tension through your middle. Alternate sides. This one is particularly challenging, so each side counts as one rep.

CIRCUIT TWO

SPLIT-STANCE LUNGE TAP TO TWIST

1. Adopt a split stance with one foot 90cm (3ft) in front of the other. Take your arms in a wide T-shape in line with your shoulders and tuck in your tailbone to help promote balance through deep-core engagement.
2. Tap the opposite hand to the inside of the front foot as you drop into a lunge, then push through the front heel to extend the leg and open the opposite hand into a gentle twist. This will strengthen the glutes and quads while promoting hip stability and thoracic spine awareness.

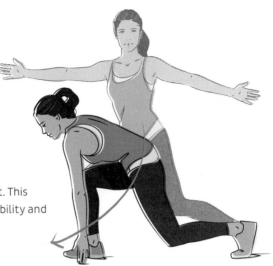

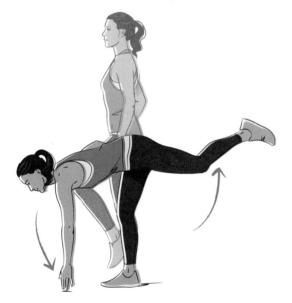

SINGLE-LEG DEADLIFT

1. Standing on the same leg you just had in front, hover the opposite foot and hinge from the hip to fold forwards. Try to keep both hips level and square to the front or to the floor throughout.
2. Focus on the hamstring of the grounded leg to stand. You can touch the floor or lower by 30–60cm (1–2ft), only going as far as you can while maintaining your balance and returning to standing upright without wobbling.

SINGLE-LEG PISTOL SQUAT

1. Find a bench, chair or platform that is roughly level with your knees when you sit. Stand with your back to it, balancing on the same working leg while floating the opposite foot just off the floor.
2. Slowly drop your bum back and lower yourself to the bench. Make sure your knee tracks over the toe – you'll probably have to imagine you're gently rotating it out in order to do so.
3. Without fully resting your seat on the bench, return to standing on one leg, keeping the weight in the heel to avoid swinging or using momentum.

The Energiser

45 mins

Movement is a powerful form of therapy, and that's particularly true in the early stages of pregnancy, when your growing baby's demands rely so heavily on your own energy stores. This month's resistance workout has two main objectives: to bank maximum energy for both you and baby by boosting blood flow and nutrient delivery; and to keep your heart above your hips so your newly dilated blood vessels can support those demands as efficiently as possible.

Perform three sets of each glute activator as an extension to the warm-up (page 30). It's important to spend time engaging the muscles that support the lower back, as this month's primary strength segment uses full-body compound movements that will require good muscle awareness. Do all five exercises of the kettlebell circuit consecutively, for a total of four rounds. The cool-down (page 32) is a great place to stretch and find a moment of well-deserved stillness.

Mindful Mamas
Choose a light kettlebell that allows you to complete twelve to fifteen reps of each exercise comfortably.

Tandem Athletes
Choose a medium to heavy kettlebell that allows you to complete eight to twelve reps of each exercise, ensuring the final few reps of each exercise feel challenging.

GLUTE ACTIVATORS

RESISTANCE LOOP BIRD DOG

1. With a resistance loop just above your knees, come to all fours with a flat back and a scooped belly button.
2. Simultaneously reach your opposite arm and leg off the floor until your hand is in line with your shoulder and your foot is in line with your hip.
3. Check your lower back is still flat at the top of the movement. If you're compromising your basic position, try a loop with less resistance. You should primarily feel the glutes and core working, with gentle tension through the back of the shoulder and down the lumbar spine.
4. Do all your reps on one side before switching. That's one set.

Equipment

Medium kettlebell (6–10kg/13–22lb)

Resistance loop

Swiss ball

RESISTANCE LOOP CLAMSHELL

1. Keeping the loop above your knees, lie on your side with your knees bent and your heels in line with your hips. You can rest on your elbow or forearm.
2. Without rolling your top hip backwards, lift the top knee until you feel a squeeze in the side of your hip. Slowly lower.
3. Do all your reps on one side before switching. That's one set.

Modification: If that felt very easy, try elevating both heels off the floor for an advanced variation.

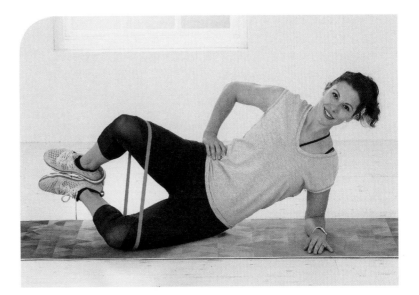

RESISTANCE LOOP LEG EXTENSION

1. Assume the same starting position as the clamshell above, but move the loop around the middle of each foot. Rest on your elbow and hip, gently pulling the side of your body away from the floor.
2. Lifting the top foot slightly, flex your heel and push the leg straight out against the resistance of the loop. You should feel this in the middle of your glute.
3. Do all the reps on one side of your body before switching. That's one set.

Modification: If that felt very easy, try lifting into a more active side plank, anchoring between your elbow and your knee.

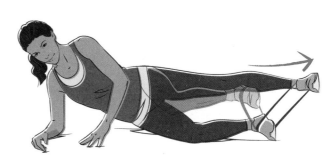

KETTLEBELL CIRCUIT

KETTLEBELL CLEAN & PRESS

1. Holding a kettlebell with your palm facing you, gently bend in the knees and powerfully pull the kettlebell up alongside your body. To adopt 'clean' position, flick your wrist at shoulder height so the palm faces forward.
2. Soften once again in the knees and use the extension of your legs, along with constant tension in your core, to press the kettlebell towards the sky. Your hand should be directly above your shoulder.
3. Reverse the movement step by step and lower into a soft squat to switch hands. Working both sides makes one rep.

Modification: If this is too challenging on the wrists, you can use a dumbbell instead of a kettlebell to master the technique first.

KETTLEBELL LUNGE

1. Holding the kettlebell in your right hand, take your left leg back and lower into a lunge. Simultaneously pass the kettlebell under your right knee and collect it with your left hand.
2. Drive the left foot in to return to standing.
3. Take the right leg back and pass the kettlebell under the left knee. That's one rep. Keep the hips neatly tucked and pelvis beneath the rib cage throughout.

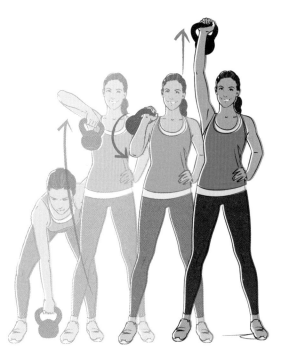

KETTLEBELL SWINGS

1. In a hip-width stance, hold a kettlebell between your legs and hinge at the hips to let it fall naturally behind you.
2. Explosively pushing your hips forward, allow the bell to swing to shoulder level. Squeeze your glutes so your spine is strong and straight at the top.
3. Make sure you are folding from the hips and not bending at the knees to generate the movement. If a kettlebell swing looks like a squat, it means you are using your thighs and your arms, but you should feel it only in your glutes. This is a powerful, dynamic movement and a great way to add low-impact cardio to your prenatal weight training.

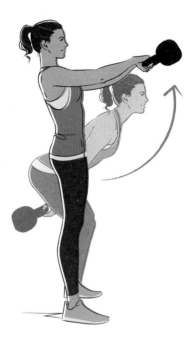

KETTLEBELL PULLOVERS

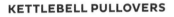

1. Resting your middle back on a bench, sofa or Swiss ball, hold a kettlebell with straight arms, maintaining a gentle bend in the elbows.
2. Keep your posterior chain engaged, drawing your navel to your spine and pushing your glutes forward so you have constant tension through your torso.
3. Moving only your arms, sweep your elbows back and in line with your ears.
4. Squeeze your lats and your chest to bring the kettlebell back in line with your chest. This will isometrically work your core and dynamically strengthen your chest and side body.

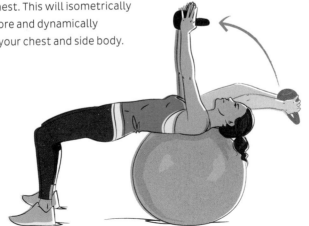

ELEVATED PLANK ROW

1. Assume an elevated plank position with your feet on the floor and your hands on a bench or sofa so your body forms a ramp-like angle.
2. Hold a kettlebell in one hand and gently absorb your weight in the other hand. Row your elbow into the side of your body, squeezing your shoulder blades together and simultaneously rolling the hip forwards to keep it square.
3. This move hits a lot of muscles at once – your deep core, your middle back and even the fronts of your thighs. Do all your reps on one side before switching to the other.

Month Three Wellness Agenda

Whether you feel just a bit bloated or you're smiling down on the first signs of a blossoming belly, it's time to master the art of engaging your deep-core muscles to keep them strong and connected as they stretch to accommodate your growing baby.

- Consolidate key movements you've learned into full-body compound exercises that continue to challenge and excite you.

- Focus on maintaining constant, gentle tension in your core to maintain safe alignment during every exercise.

- Strengthen the joints by working mindfully in different directions, making sure the knees and hips remain stable for all the demands of your active, everyday life.

- Choose exercise modifications that keep your head above your heart if you are still feeling the light-headed effects of vascular underfill.

BUCKWHEAT CHIA PIZZA

Serves Two

120g (4½oz) chickpeas
(drained)
150g (5½oz) courgette, sliced
into long, thin strips
15 tbsp buckwheat flour
1 avocado, peeled, de-stoned
and finely sliced
1 garlic clove, finely chopped
1 red onion, thinly sliced
2 tbsp balsamic vinegar
2 tbsp chia seeds
40g (1½oz) rocket
4 tsp oil
Medium handful of fresh
basil, finely sliced

639 calories · 86g carbs · 27g fat ·
21g protein

This simple recipe uses superfood chia seeds, a great source of dairy-free calcium to promote baby's bone development.

1. Preheat the oven to 200C / gas mark 6 and line two baking sheets with baking parchment. In a bowl, mix the chia seeds with 6 tbsp cold water and leave for 5 mins.
2. Mix the buckwheat flour with the chia mix, a pinch of sea salt and 8 tbsp cold water to form a soft dough. Halve the dough and spread out into a pizza shape (approx. 15cm (6in) diameter) on one of the prepared baking sheets. Repeat with the remaining dough. Place the pizzas in the oven for 15 mins.
3. Meanwhile, drain the chickpeas then add to a bowl with the garlic, 2 tsp oil and 2 tbsp cold water, then season. Mash with a potato masher until crushed, then stir the basil into the hummus mix.
4. In a frying pan over a medium heat, add 1 tsp oil and fry the onion for 5 mins. Add half of the balsamic vinegar and cook for a further 3 mins.
5. Drizzle the courgette strips with 1 tsp oil. Heat griddle pan on a medium heat and cook the courgette for 2-3 mins each side.
6. To serve, place each pizza on a warm plate. Spread over the hummus and top with the courgette, onions and avocado. Finish with a drizzle of the remaining balsamic vinegar and serve with rocket alongside.

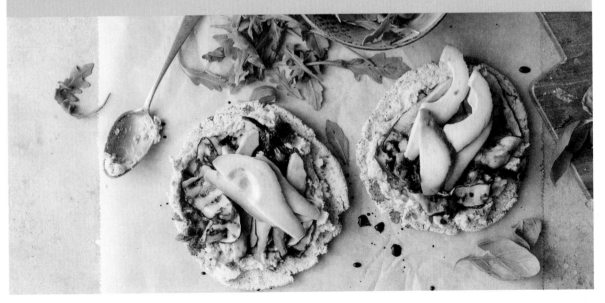

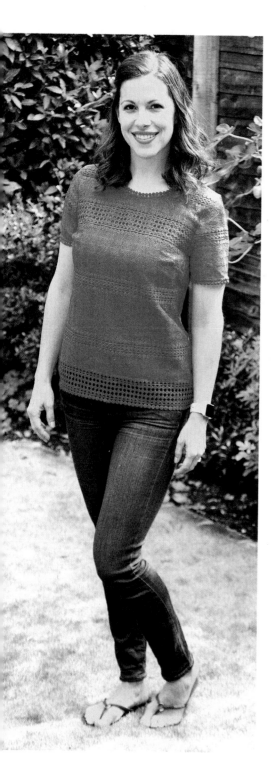

What is Happening to Your Body?

WHAT?

My philosophy on calorie counting remains unchanged for pregnancy – namely, I don't recommend it. You'll hear a few different theories about how many extra calories you need at different stages of pregnancy. But just like people who aren't pregnant (perhaps even more so), expecting mums are all completely unique, and so, too, are their nutritional needs (see page 16 for nutritional guidelines). By the end of the first trimester, around 2kg (4½lb) of extra weight gain is considered healthy.

WHY?

At this stage, baby is making up only a very small amount of your weight gain – the majority of it is extra blood volume and water weight. You may feel that most of that weight has been distributed to your chest, which is probably still the only visible evidence of your pregnancy. If you are still feeling very nauseous or are vomiting frequently, it is possible to lose a little weight in the first trimester. Try not to worry too much if this is the case. The biggest share of healthy weight gain will come after week twenty, and as hCG finally levels off around week twelve, your morning sickness is likely to subside by the end of the month.

SO WHAT?

If your first trimester has made biscuits far more tempting than wholegrains, know that your appetite and cravings are likely to look more familiar soon. Be mindful that putting on unnecessary extra kilos can impact your posture even more than the extra demands of pregnancy, and gaining a healthy amount of weight will make it far easier to get moving again as a new mum. However, if you're exercising a few times a week and eating small, frequent meals with a good balance of proteins, carbs and healthy fats, your weight gain should remain on track whether you watch the scales or not.

What is Happening to Your Baby?

BENEATH THE BUMP

There's no right or wrong time to start showing. Every woman's body changes at a different rate during pregnancy, so avoid comparing yourself to others. Regardless of what's happening on the outside, there is certainly plenty taking place on the inside.

Your juicy little raspberry becomes a rather plump plum up to 10cm (4in) long, with a host of new features including teeth buds, hair follicles, finger- and toenails and even genitals. It's not possible to tell the sex of your baby by ultrasound until at least fifteen weeks, but you can elect to have a twelve-week blood test that gives you ample information about the health of your baby, including the option to learn if it's a girl or boy, should you wish.

This month marks the completion of baby's home in your womb. The placenta is now fully developed and will begin to take over the task of primary pregnancy hormone production, plus the transfer of nourishment to your baby via the umbilical cord. As these systems stabilise, you'll also get a break from any morning sickness you've experienced.

BUILDING AN ATHLETE

Baby's spine begins a serious growth spurt this month, with the skeleton primarily made up of cartilage that will harden into bone over time. In fact, this process continues well into your child's twenties, so continue taking folic acid to establish strong foundations.

Upping your calcium intake during pregnancy will also help to support your baby's bone development. The richest source is dairy, so include plenty of cow's milk, yoghurt and pregnancy-safe cheeses in your diet. If you are lactose intolerant or need to avoid dairy for any reason, chia seeds are a great alternative. Three tablespoons provide the calcium equivalent of a glass of milk. As an added bonus, chia seeds' high fibre content will help to prevent constipation, which is common during pregnancy because progesterone relaxes the smooth muscle of your digestive tract.

BABY PBs

If your heart is feeling particularly full for the life within, know that baby's heart is full too, as it completes its development and establishes a healthy resting heart rate three times faster than your own.

As baby's skeleton becomes increasingly functional, baby will enjoy putting his or her new limbs to use. You won't feel those punches and kicks just yet, but your twelve-week scan will show baby moving comfortably around his or her cosy nest.

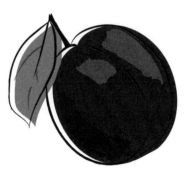

Fit to Adapt

40 mins

If pregnancy and motherhood teach you anything, it's how to adapt. Month three's bodyweight workout is all about equipping your body with the strength, balance and stability to tackle the changes coming its way. You'll incorporate plenty of full-body lateral movements to strengthen the joints in every direction, and work your obliques so they continue to support your spine while your deep core and 'six-pack' muscles get gradually stretched in the coming months.

After your warm-up (page 30), challenge yourself to complete the pyramid superset as quickly as you can while maintaining perfect form. Then perform three rounds of circuit one followed by three of circuit two – follow the format recommended for your chosen level or build from Mindful Mama to Tandem Athlete throughout the month. Always finish with the cool-down (page 32).

Mindful Mamas
Complete twelve reps of each exercise in circuits one and two. For circuit one, do the exercises on each side to make up one round.

Tandem Athletes
Perform twelve reps of the exercises in circuits one and two. For circuit one, perform three rounds on one side, before repeating on the other side.

PYRAMID SUPERSET

Complete four rounds of the following superset, following the ascending and descending repetition pyramid shown in the circle, right. Challenge yourself to complete the pyramid in under ten minutes.

ROUND 1: 8 LP – 20 SL
ROUND 2: 12 LP – 16 SL
ROUND 3: 16 LP – 12 SL
ROUND 4: 20 LP – 8 SL

LATERAL PRESS-UPS (LP)

1. Assume a high plank position on the floor – or on a raised platform if you feel any light-headedness due to sudden position changes.
2. Allow your hands to meet in line with your chest, then step one hand out to the side beyond the shoulder and lower into an offset press-up.
3. Bring the hands back together as you extend your arm and repeat to the other side. Each side counts towards your reps.

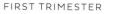

SIDE LUNGES (SL)

1. Standing in a neutral position, take a big step out to the side, keeping the inside edges of your feet parallel.
2. Melt your hip over your heel, keeping the grounded leg straight.
3. Dynamically push off the floor and return to centre. As with the press-ups, alternate sides and count each side as a rep.

CIRCUIT ONE

SUMO SQUAT TO LATERAL LEG LIFT

1. Assume a sumo squat position with your feet wider than your hips and your toes turned out to forty-five degrees.
2. Drop into a low squat, then transfer your weight into one leg as you come to stand and laterally extend the other leg to the side.
3. Both legs are working, but you should feel an extra squeeze in the glute of the extending leg.

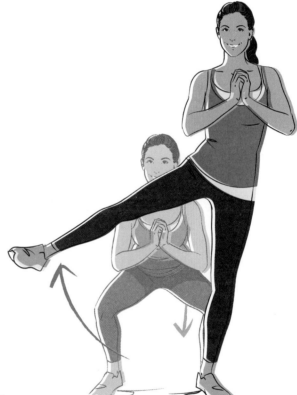

STATIC LUNGE KNEE DRIVE

1. Placing the extending leg from the squat in front, drop into your lowest lunge position.
2. Without lifting your front thigh or allowing your knee to roll in, drive the back leg from lunge position to squat position and back again.
3. Minimise momentum and keep your hips rolling forward. This one should build a nice heat in the thigh and glutes of the front leg.

PIGEON BRIDGE

1. Combine a lovely hip stretch with more glute strengthening. Bring the same working leg as above into a pigeon position, folding the opposite leg behind you so your legs form a zigzag.
2. Squeezing your front glutes, lift your bum off your heels and dynamically push your hips up into a high kneeling position. Your back should stay straight and your front hip should feel a stretch at the top.
3. Resist momentum and return slowly to the floor. Try to keep both hips pointing forward to make the most of this movement. The hip flexor will contract and lengthen, helping to counteract any overstretching that can take place as your bump pulls your hips forward later in pregnancy.

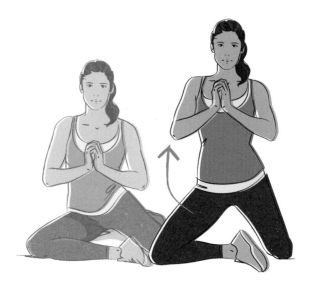

CIRCUIT TWO

BIRD DOG COUNTER SWEEP

1. From an all-fours position, complete a bird dog with your left arm and right leg reaching up and away simultaneously.
2. At the top of the movement, send your arm out to the left and your leg out to the right. Try to keep your chest and hips square to the floor throughout, and your arm and leg in line with your torso.
3. Slowly reverse the steps and return to all fours. One side is one rep. Alternate sides.

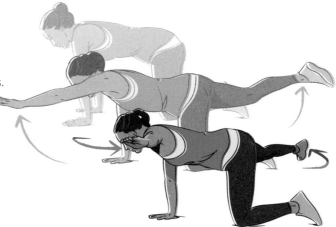

SIDE PLANK MERMAID

1. In a three-quarter or full forearm-supported side plank, slowly sink your lower hip to the floor and keep your top arm resting on your hip.
2. Squeezing your obliques, slowly peel your waist away from the floor and reach your top arm overhead so your elbow meets your ear.
3. Repeat all reps on one side before switching, and make sure that the hips remain stacked on both sides.

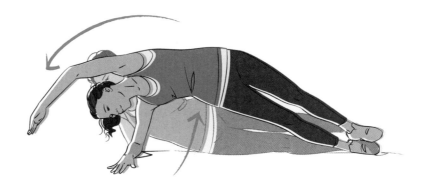

AB RECLINERS

1. In a seated position with your knees gently bent in front of you, create a soft C curve with your spine as you roll your shoulders back, roughly forty-five degrees to the floor.
2. Holding this position, sweep your arms overhead so your elbows are in line with your ears. Pause for a second at the top – you'll know the movement is working if you feel a tremble deep within your core.
3. Lower your arms back to the start.

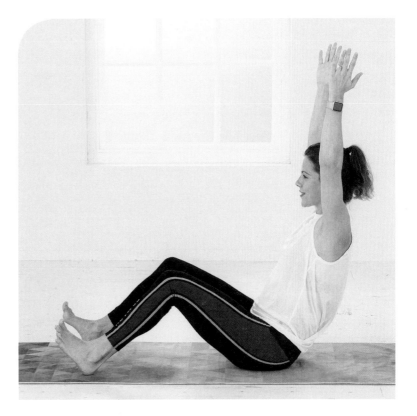

Bell & The Bump

40 mins

This month's resistance workout consolidates key movements you've learned into full-body compound exercises. You'll also get invaluable practice maintaining safe and consistent tension in your core while isolating muscles in the upper body. As your abdominals stretch, it's important you know how to engage them properly to avoid over-straining and separation; now is the time to master this skill.

After your warm-up (page 30), work through all five exercises of the kettlebell circuit in quick succession, resting only when you've completed a round. Repeat for a total of four rounds. For a fun finale that aids a deeper connection between the core and the glutes, set a timer and complete both exercises of the resistance band superset for sixty seconds, then forty-five seconds, then thirty seconds each. You may want to hang out in pigeon a little longer as you wrap up with the cool-down (page 32).

Mindful Mamas

Choose a light kettlebell that allows you to complete twelve to fourteen reps of each exercise in the kettlebell circuit. Add an optional rest period between the three rounds of the resistance band superset – no longer than the length of each exercise in the round.

Tandem Athletes

Choose a medium to heavy kettlebell that allows you to complete eight to ten reps of each exercise in the kettlebell circuit, ensuring the final reps of each exercise are challenging. Aim to complete the resistance band superset with minimum rest between rounds – no more than half the duration of each exercise.

Equipment

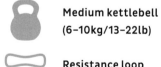

Medium kettlebell
(6–10kg/13–22lb)

Resistance loop

KETTLEBELL CIRCUIT

SQUAT CLEAN & LUNGE PRESS

1. This move layers the dynamic lunge press of month one with the clean & press of month two (see pages 45 and 56). Choose a lighter kettlebell or dumbbell to master the more complex movement.
2. Squat low and drive explosively through your heels as you pull the kettlebell up your body and flick your wrist to face forward at the top.
3. Now drop the opposite leg back into a reverse lunge as you simultaneously press the kettlebell up in line with your shoulder. Do all your reps on the same side before switching arms and legs.

Modification: If you feel light-headed, remove the shoulder press and keep the hand in clean position while you lunge.

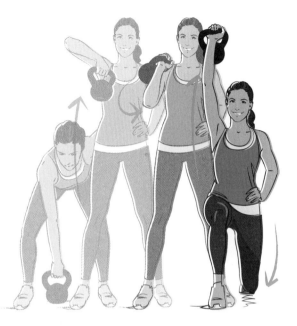

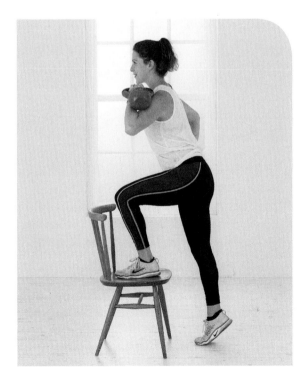

STEP-UP

1. Using a bench or platform that is ideally knee height or slightly higher, place one foot on the platform and drive through the foot to extend the raised leg.
2. Slowly step back down, without letting the knee roll in. Continue all your reps on one side before switching. Avoid using the bottom leg to help you lift away from the floor.
3. You can keep a kettlebell in clean position above the working leg, or rest it alongside your hip on the same side. If you begin to use momentum to complete your reps, remove the kettlebell and focus on good form first.

HIGH ROW

1. Split your stance and support one hand on either the knee of the front leg or on a raised platform, keeping your back flat and hips square.
2. Holding a kettlebell in your other hand, draw your elbow out to the side and in line with your shoulder.
3. Think about pulling the tops of your shoulders away from your ears so you feel the squeeze in your upper back. Complete all your reps on one side before switching.

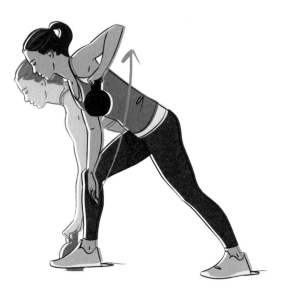

PLANK PULL-THROUGHS

1. Assume an elevated plank position with your feet on the floor and your hands on a bench or sofa so your body forms a ramp-like angle.

2. Place a kettlebell just behind and outside of your left hand. Without rolling your hips, weave your right arm under your left to pick up the kettlebell and pull it to the same position outside your right hand. Both sides make up one rep.

3. This move will work your deep core and the sides of the back at once.

Modification: Lower the knees into a three-quarter plank position if you require more lumbar support or pelvic stability.

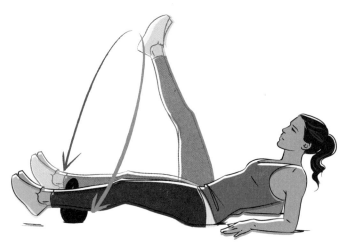

LEG CIRCLES

1. Place the kettlebell so that it sits where your ankles would be in a seated position with your legs outstretched.
2. Lying on your back, or resting on your forearms if you feel dizzy on your back, maintain a neutral spine and active core as you raise your legs seventy-five to ninety degrees from the ground.
3. Draw a slow semicircle to the left and down to the kettlebell, then reverse the movement back to the top. Keep your tailbone gently tucked and your navel pulled to avoid any doming in your abdomen.
4. Mindful Mamas, count each side as one rep. Tandem Athletes, count both sides as one rep.

RESISTANCE BAND SUPERSET

WALL-SQUAT ABDUCTION

1. Standing with your back against a wall, place a resistance loop above your knees and slide down the wall so your knees are bent to ninety degrees.
2. Holding this static squat position, gently pulse your knees out to the sides against the resistance of the loop. You should feel your gluteus medius – the sides of your bum.
3. Resist allowing your knees to fall in on themselves, only moving them from a start position above your ankles and a finish position outside your ankles.

SINGLE-LEG PLANK JACKS

1. Keep the loop in place and assume a high plank position (use a raised surface if you feel light-headed).
2. Without rolling your hips, step one leg about 15cm (6in) to one side, then back through centre before switching sides. That's one rep.
3. The movement should come from your gluteus medius – the part of your hips that was feeling rather fiery during your wall-squat abduction.

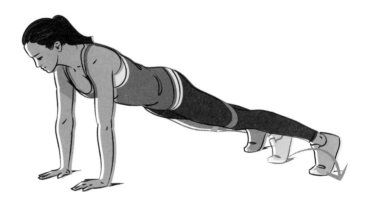

A Word on Miscarriage

It's a sad reality that an estimated one in four pregnancies results in miscarriage, seventy-five per cent of which occur in the first trimester. Miscarriages are not a result of maternal mistakes, but are caused by reasons that remain largely unknown.

What we do know is that there is nothing you can do to cause miscarriage – 80% are associated with chromosomal abnormalities in the baby. It's essential you do not live in fear during the early weeks of your pregnancy, or blame yourself if your pregnancy proves unviable. While particularly tragic for expecting mums, miscarriage is nature's way of ensuring babies have the best possible prospects when they reach full term. If you have previously experienced a miscarriage, know that the vast majority of women go on to have healthy babies, so approach your current pregnancy with optimism.

If this is your first pregnancy, exercise can help you to overcome any anxiety you may feel about miscarriage. In fact, a slate of new studies show that women with a strong foundation in fitness can maintain much the same intensity of exercise in early pregnancy, with no extra risk to maternal or fetal health.

Always call your GP or midwife if you experience vaginal bleeding, pain or a loss of pregnancy symptoms that cause you to feel concerned. There are a few proactive measures you can take to create the healthiest possible home for a viable baby:

- Reduce caffeine intake to less than 200mg per day (roughly one cup of filter coffee, two shots of espresso or two mugs of tea)

- Abstain from smoking

- Abstain from alcohol

- Keep cool while you exercise – frequent rest and hydration breaks can help ease feelings of nausea in the first trimester

- Talk to your GP or midwife if you have any pre-existing health issues such as diabetes, high blood pressure or under- or overactive thyroid activity that may require additional monitoring during pregnancy. Always seek advice about managing these conditions before beginning a new exercise regime.

- If you are diagnosed with a weak cervix, avoid strenuous exercise or adhere to the activity levels your GP or midwife advises.

TALK MENTAL HEALTH

If early pregnancy makes you feel tingly with nerves rather than tingly with excitement, know that you're not alone. According to new research published in 2018, one-quarter of women surveyed admitted to suffering mental health problems during pregnancy. If you're keeping your pregnancy a private affair until you reach the twelve-week milestone, prioritise time with your partner or family during this tentative period. Whether you feel like being intimate or not, carving out quality time to talk, cuddle or enjoy a shared activity every week will allow you to open up about your feelings and boost oxytocin levels – the love hormone that can help to promote mental well-being. If your anxiety becomes too much to handle with support from your partner, family or friends, ask your GP or midwife to signpost you to a women's health counsellor who can help.

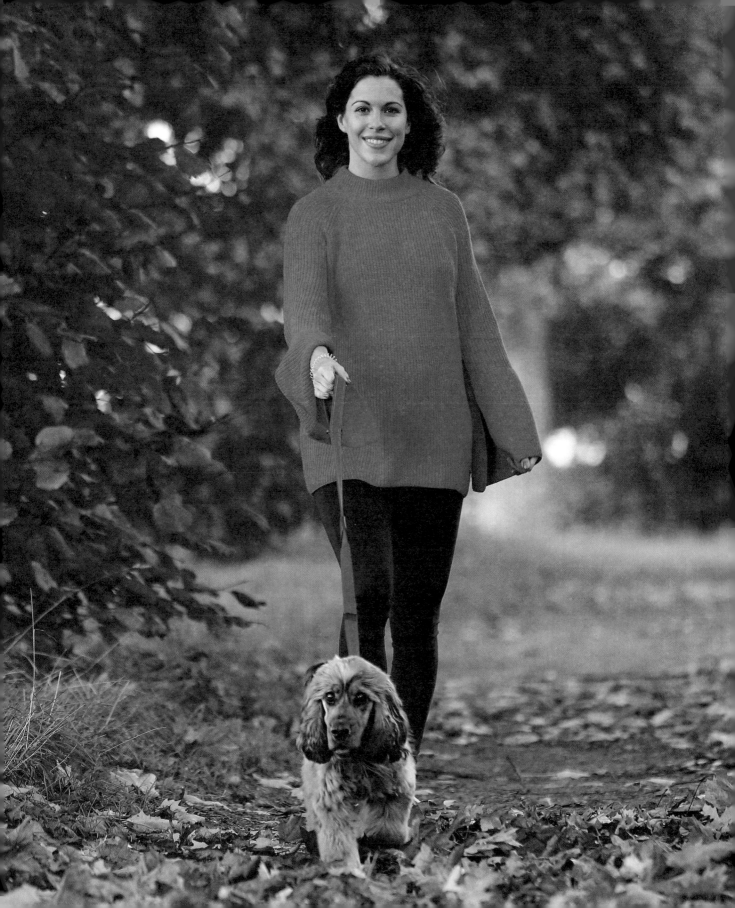

SECOND TRIMESTER

—

13–27 WEEKS

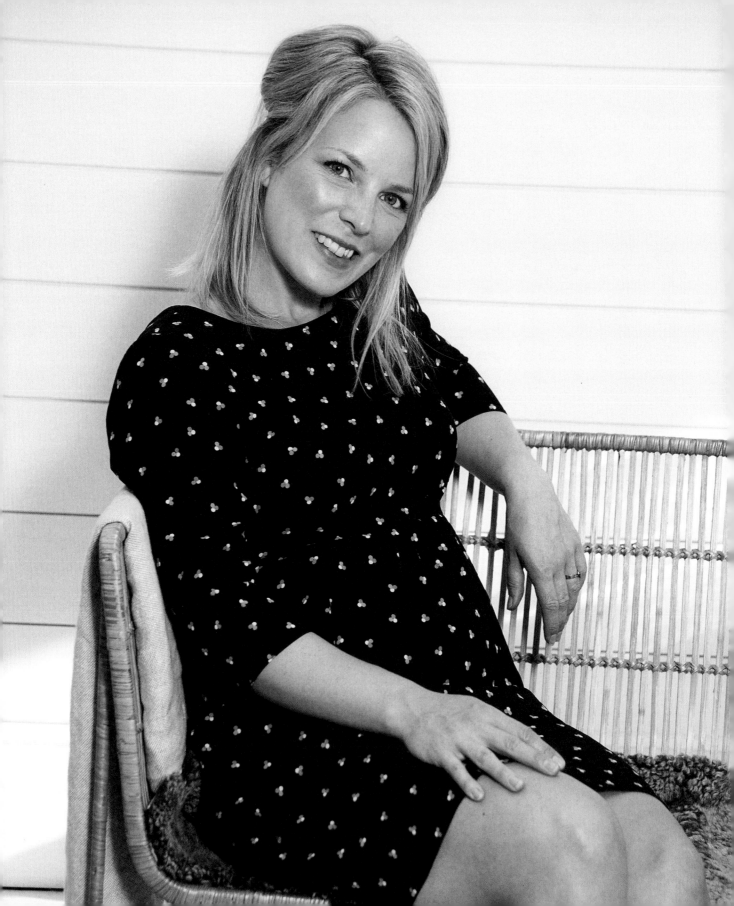

Training for Two

Go on and breathe a little sigh of relief. The hormones that may have turned your world upside down in the first three months are now to thank for your second trimester pregnancy glow. Add the joy of sharing and celebrating your news, exciting firsts like baby's early movements and an increasingly evident bump (which helpfully moves up and off your bladder).

If a tough first trimester sidelined your intentions for an active pregnancy, you can also look forward to enjoying exercise again. You can adopt the *MBB* approach to exercise at any stage of your pregnancy. Rather than jumping straight into the workouts for your current month, practise the month one workouts (see pages 38–45) – which are safe for every stage of pregnancy – for a week or two until you feel confident with the foundational movements. Then join in with the month-by-month workouts relevant to you.

As you regain your sense of self, your choices now can have a powerful effect on your baby's senses in and out of the womb. If you find yourself having to decide between filling up on salmon fillets or tucking into giant tubs of ice cream during pregnancy, there is one fascinating study that is worth bearing in mind. When it comes to making healthier dietary choices, researchers have demonstrated that weaning babies react more positively to the flavours their mothers prioritised during pregnancy. It certainly gives new meaning to the phrase 'eating for two'.

Your Changing Body

If the reality of your pregnancy hasn't quite hit, a quick look beneath your blooming bump will give you new respect for your body. As fast as your body is changing, baby is evolving more rapidly still. Keeping up with your children will be your greatest ever motivation to stay fit. Goodbye #fitspo, hello #familyspo.

BRAIN

Your celebratory arrival at the second trimester is likely to cause a surge of the happiness hormone serotonin. Revel in it! Nervous jitters around the twenty-week mark could arise from higher cortisol levels if the anomaly scan causes you apprehension. Listen to your body and move slowly and mindfully during workouts if you feel any anxiety. Exercise should be an outlet, not an added stress.

STOMACH

As your appetite returns, intense cravings may be your body's way of correcting subtle nutrient deficiencies common in pregnancy. Hankering for red meat? Could be your red blood cells demanding more iron. Pickles calling out to you? Increased blood volume means higher sodium requirements, making salty foods extra tempting.

HEART

As your blood volume catches up and fills your newly dilated blood vessels, any palpitations you may have experienced should begin to ease. You may feel less breathless during workouts and require less rest. Enjoy it, as increasing pressure from your bump on your diaphragm will change the game again soon enough.

BREASTS

Your breasts will continue to grow during this trimester, but you may notice them less as your bump expands beneath them. They will also become less sensitive as the pregnancy hormones level off. If you're concerned about stretch marks, an oil rich in omega and vitamin E can help to support the skin's natural elasticity.

OVARIES

The ovaries become the secondary site of pregnancy hormone production in the second and third trimesters, with much more support from the placenta. Stable yet elevated hormone levels will increase natural oil production – cue glowing skin and shiny hair.

PLACENTA

Now a very busy site of hormone production and nutrient transfer to your baby, the placenta is the kitchen of the womb. Maintaining healthy blood flow with regular exercise will support it in its role as personal chef to your baby.

BLADDER

As your bump takes shape and lifts away from your pelvis, your bladder gets a little relief. However, staying adequately hydrated during pregnancy should still require you to take frequent loo breaks.

BLOOD VESSELS

As your blood volume continues to increase, symptoms of vascular underfill should begin to subside. This increased blood volume, paired with dilated vessels, explains why pooling blood and varicose veins are common in pregnancy. You can help to prevent them by regularly elevating your feet and frequently changing from seated to standing positions to improve circulation.

Beginnings & Endings

Some of the biggest prenatal changes you'll experience take place in the second trimester, so it's more important than ever that you mentally clock in and out of your workouts. The following warm-up will help you engage key supporting muscles that will protect you as your centre of gravity changes. The cool-down emphasises length in the most compromised muscles of pregnancy.

SECOND TRIMESTER WARM-UP

Perform each of the following five exercises once through. Aim to spend roughly one minute on each exercise, slowing down and using the breath to release tension in the hips, open the shoulders, engage the core and find safe spinal alignment. If your hips, IT band, hamstrings, latissimus dorsi (lats) or upper back feel particularly tight, spend a few moments foam rolling these muscles before your warm-up (see page 107).

ROTATING ALL FOURS

1. On all fours, with your shoulders over your hands and your hips over your knees, gently rotate your body to the right, back, left and forward.
2. Try five slow circles followed by five fast circles, looking to release any tension through the back and gently drawing in the navel to connect with the core muscles.
3. Once you've completed ten reps in one direction, reverse and repeat ten reps in the opposite direction.

PLANK DOWN-DOG SHIFTERS

1. Assume a high plank position with a gentle bend in your elbows, shoulders rolling away from the earth and a gentle upward pull from your kneecaps to your neckline.
2. As you exhale, roll onto the balls of your feet and send your hips high, pushing away from your hands. Roll your elbows gently in so you work through the biceps as well as the shoulders. At the top of the position, soften your heels towards the floor and hold.
3. As you inhale, roll back to tiptoes and slowly transfer your shoulders over your hands, reconnecting and lifting through the front of the body. Continue moving with your breath for ten reps.

x10

TICK-TOCK LEGS

1. In a supine position with your knees bent, feet hip-width apart and arms extended to the sides, gently allow both knees to fall to the left. Hold for moment, feeling a release in the left hip flexor. Repeat to the right – that's one rep. Do ten.
2. Try to exhale as you move into the stretch and inhale as you return through the centre. Make sure your torso remains connected to the floor, with just the legs moving.

Modification: When you reach the five-month mark, modify by elevating your heart above your hips. Resting your shoulder blades on a wide yoga block or a pillow should do the trick.

x10

SIDE-LYING THORACIC MOBILISERS

1. Lie on your side with your knees bent and stacked, your arms extended on the floor in front of you and palms touching and in line with heart centre.
2. Minimising rotation in your top hip, roll the top shoulder open and allow the back of your hand to tap the floor behind you. You should feel a dynamic stretch in your mid-back.
3. Complete ten reps on one side, then switch.

x10

GODDESS SQUAT SHOULDER SHIMMIES

1. Assume a wide squat with your toes turned out, weight in your heels and your hands gently resting inside your knees. If it's comfortable, lower your hips to ninety degrees. If you have any pelvic discomfort, hips above knees is absolutely fine.
2. While stabilising your lower body, rotate one shoulder down and frame your chest central to the opposite leg. Feel the stretch down the side of your body.
3. Alternate sides to complete the rep, moving into the stretch on the exhale and through centre on the inhale.

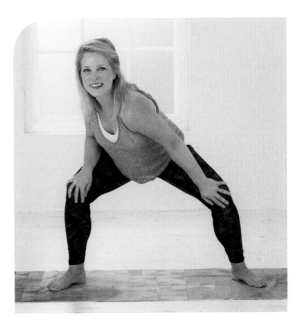

SECOND TRIMESTER COOL-DOWN

Hold each of these stretches for at least as long as instructed, using each exhale to release more tension. Rather than bouncing in a position, let the lengthened muscle soften within the hold. If you feel particularly constricted, simply tune in to your body and invest more time in the relevant stretch, or try multiple sets of the same stretch and take note of any changes.

HALF-SPLIT HAMSTRING STRETCH

1. From a high kneeling position, extend one foot in front of you and flex your toes to the sky. If you feel the stretch in your back leg, stay here.
2. If you need a deeper stretch, use your inhale to lengthen through the spine and exhale to fold your chest over your leg. Avoid rounding through your upper back.
3. Hold for five to eight breaths on both sides.

ALL-FOURS BOW STRETCH

1. From all fours, extend your right arm and left leg. Keep your navel drawn in to avoid collapsing in the lower back. This is your basic position.
2. If you can maintain this connection, bend your left knee and reach back with your right hand to grab the inside of your left foot. Gently kick into your hand and open through your chest to create a subtle bow-like shape through your back.
3. If you feel any discomfort, regress to the basic position and focus on maximising the distance between your fingertips and your toes. Hold for five to eight breaths, then switch sides.

PIGEON STRETCH

1. From all fours, fold your right shin across your body and allow the left thigh to soften to the floor behind you.
2. Simultaneously soften into both hips, encouraging your right hip towards the floor and your left hip towards your right foot.
3. Keep this movement static and enjoy a few deep breaths, or make it dynamic and alternate between rounding and opening your shoulders to massage your middle back. Repeat on the other side.

WIDE-LEG CHILD'S POSE

1. From kneeling, shimmy your knees as far beyond hip-width apart as possible, creating space in your pelvis without feeling discomfort. From here, sink your hips over your heels and stretch your fingertips in front of you.

2. Allow your head to be heavy and your forehead to rest on the floor. This is a nice place to rest a little longer and focus on your breath.

3. Stay for as long as feels good, melting deeper into your heels with each exhale and stretching further through the fingertips with each inhale.

THREAD THE NEEDLE THORACIC STRETCH

1. Return to all fours. Shifting your weight into your left hand, and minimising rotation in your right hip, open through the right shoulder and reach your fingertips to the sky. Accompany this movement with your inhale.

2. As you exhale, thread your right arm under your left armpit and allow the back of the shoulder to rest on the floor. Repeat five to eight times on one side before switching to the other side.

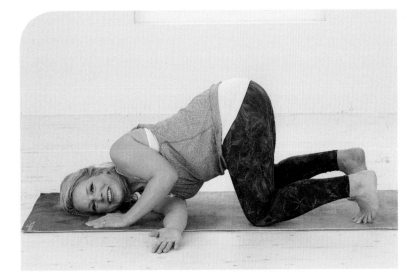

Month Four Wellness Agenda

As you skip into the first month of trimester two, channel your newfound energy into moving more regularly and mindfully. There are some new exercise limitations around the corner, but for now most movement patterns are safe and you still have a vast variety of exercises available to you.

- If you enjoy impact activities like running, you can continue to do so. Try to incorporate mindful breathing and pelvic floor integration (see page 28) in order to strengthen these key support muscles.

- While you may find you need less rest during your workouts, carve out time after or outside of workouts to stretch and tune in to subtle changes in your body.

- If repetitive movements like walking, jogging or cycling have an adverse effect on round ligament pain, prioritise strength training and incorporate a variety of movement patterns in your workouts.

- Practise changing position from standing, sitting and kneeling frequently – during and outside of your workouts – in order to promote good circulation.

- To improve whole-body balance, advance your workout routine with more unilateral exercises (moving one leg or arm at a time), which require you to engage from your centre.

- Personalise and take charge of your workouts, responding to any niggles that come up by substituting or removing exercises that feel uncomfortable. Remember that the workouts in this book are a guideline and that every body and every pregnancy is unique.

SPINACH FALAFELS WITH ZINGY KALE SALAD

Serves Two

This vegetarian dish combines pulses and nuts to make up a complete protein. Spinach and kale bring a powerful dose of restorative magnesium.

100g (3½oz) spinach
1/2 pomegranate
15g (½oz) creamed coconut
1 avocado
1 tbsp oil
1 tsp harissa paste
20g (¾oz) walnuts
240g (8½oz) chickpeas (drained)
2 tbsp apple cider vinegar
2 tbsp chickpea flour
80g (2¾oz) kale

557 calories · 57g carbs · 35g fat · 18g protein

1. Preheat the oven to 200C/gas mark 6 and boil a kettle.
2. Drain the chickpeas and place in bowl, mash for 1-2 mins with a potato masher or the back of a fork until all the chickpeas are crushed.
3. Place the spinach in a separate bowl. Pour over boiling water to cover and leave to wilt for 1 min. Drain the wilted spinach in a sieve and squeeze out any excess water. Finely chop.
4. Add the chopped spinach to the bowl of chickpeas with the chickpea flour, 1 tsp olive oil and 1 tbsp water. Season generously and mix well. Form the chickpea mixture into 12 balls and place on a baking tray in the oven for 15-20 mins, turning halfway through.
5. Meanwhile, to make the kale salad: finely slice the kale (removing any tough stalks); cut the pomegranate in half and remove the seeds. Peel and de-stone the avocado, then cut into small pieces. Roughly chop the walnuts. Mix all these ingredients together in a bowl, then mix in the apple cider vinegar and 1/2 tbsp oil. Season with sea salt and black pepper.
6. In a separate bowl, dissolve the creamed coconut with 30ml (1fl oz) boiling water and mix with the harissa paste.
7. Serve the falafels on two plates and drizzle over the coconut harissa sauce. Serve alongside the zingy kale salad.

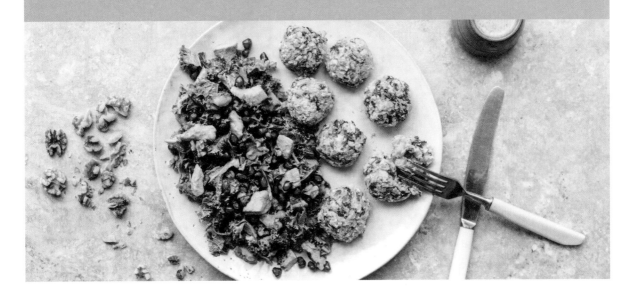

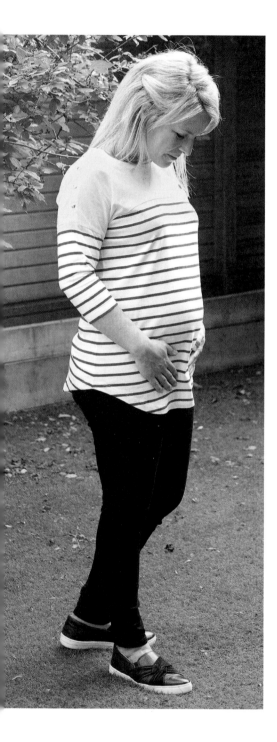

What is Happening to Your Body?

WHAT?

Soon your belly, which probably looks no more than a bit bloated, is going to expand rapidly. In preparation, supporting tissues of the uterus, known as round ligaments, may contract or spasm. If you feel jabbing pains or cramp-like sensations in your lower abdomen, this ligament activity is typically the cause and it's incredibly common around month four. Although alarming, these contractions are harmless and are essential for softening the pelvis for the later stages of pregnancy and childbirth.

WHY?

Repetitive motion is most likely to cause round ligament pain. Try to avoid rushing around; allow more time getting from A to B so you can stop for regular rests.

The relaxin hormone that enables this ligament softening is the culprit behind another common pregnancy symptom: constipation. As the digestive organs relax and become a little lazier than usual, upping fibre intake, staying hydrated and keeping active will help keep your gut moving.

SO WHAT?

This is a great time to begin moving more mindfully and enjoy slower stretches between workouts or as part of your cool-down. The *MBB* stretches will promote balance in your body, as some muscles naturally become longer and weaker, while others become shorter and tighter.

Remember, too, that you're sharing your nutrient intake with your baby, so if you do feel increased post-workout stiffness, listen to your body and respond by upping the quantity of protein in your diet. Eating extra magnesium-rich foods may also help, as the mineral is integral to protein synthesis and muscular function. Nuts and seeds are doubly effective, as they pack in plenty of magnesium while promoting your body's natural anti-inflammatory responses.

What is Happening to Your Baby?

BENEATH THE BUMP

Perhaps the most Instagrammed growth reference out there, this month your baby will graduate to the size of an avocado. His or her head is still disproportionately large – all the better to hear you with! Although it can't yet judge whether you have the X-factor, your baby can hear the muffled sound of you speaking and singing. It can even hear your heartbeat, which will remain a source of comfort as you hold him or her close following birth. Eyesight will follow suit soon; the eyes are still closed, but are now sensitive to light.

Baby's arms and legs are getting more mobile as bones and muscles continue to develop. Baby is probably sucking his or her thumb as the digits of the hands separate this month. He or she will also suck and swallow amniotic fluid, which helps to develop the lungs and trains the palate as the taste changes along with your diet.

BUILDING AN ATHLETE

If you have a sweet tooth that you'd prefer not to pass on, you have a chance now to influence your baby's rapidly developing sense of taste. By balancing sweet foods with savoury, you can actively change the taste of amniotic fluid your baby ingests in the womb. For fewer future battles over eating greens, try upping your own intake now.

BABY PBs

This month baby's circulatory system becomes fully functional, pumping an incredible 28 litres (49pts) of blood around his or her body every day. Let's chalk this one up as a PB for you too, as you're also pumping 150 per cent of your own usual reserve!

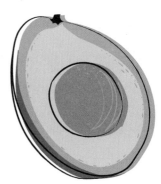

The Glow-Down

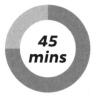

45 mins

Since you are still likely to feel much like your pre-pregnancy self this month, say hello to another high-energy bodyweight pyramid. Next month you'll start to substitute or modify supine exercises (performed lying on your back), so this is also the time to make the most of mat-based exercises that strengthen your core and glutes.

Always check in to your workout and prepare your body with the warm-up (page 78), being mindful of any niggles that may require you to modify your workout; it's always possible to substitute or remove any exercises that feel uncomfortable. Complete ten reps of each exercise, transitioning to the next consecutive move as quickly as possible until you finish on dead bugs. Rest for one minute after one full round, then return to the first exercise and complete eight reps of each exercise throughout. Continue dropping by two reps per round until your fifth and final round takes you to two reps of each exercise. Check out and stretch out with the cool-down (page 80).

Mindful Mamas

Look out for the modifications and aim to complete the workout in under forty minutes.

Tandem Athletes

Move as energetically as you can while maintaining good form and aim to complete the workout in under thirty minutes.

SQUAT TO INCHWORM

1. Stand with your feet hip-width apart. Lowering into your squat, find the floor with your hands and walk your hands out into a high plank position.
2. Reverse your walk and bend through the knees (not your back) to return to standing. That's one rep.

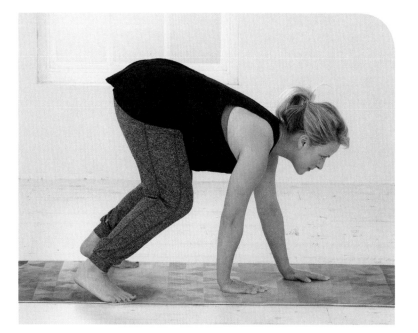

SUMO SQUAT CRUNCH

1. Widen your stance and angle your toes out to the sides. Frame your head with your elbows, keeping your chest open, as you lower into a squat.
2. As you stand, shift your weight into your left heel and draw your right knee towards your right elbow. Think knee to elbow rather than elbow to knee in order to maximise engagement of the muscles through your waist.
3. Alternate sides. Both sides make up one rep.

PRESS-UP CROSS-BODY TAP

1. Assume a high plank position, repeating all your form checks – soft elbows, rounded shoulders, quads engaged.
2. Lower into a press-up, then transfer your weight into your left hand as you come up, simultaneously driving your hips into a deep upside-down V and bringing your right hand across to your left ankle.
3. Return to your plank and repeat on the opposite side. That's one rep.

Modification: If you feel this in your lower back, complete the press-up phase on your knees, then tuck your toes to press back into the cross-body tap.

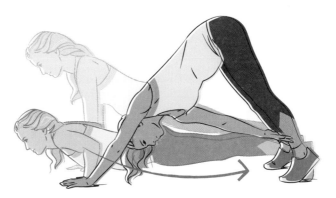

FOREARM PLANK KNEE TAPS

1. Come into a low plank, your forearms parallel to the ground and the front of your body actively drawing away from the floor.
2. Minimising rotation through the hips, lower one knee to tap the floor before returning to centre and swapping sides. That's one rep.

TRICEP DIPS

1. Using an elevated platform – a step, chair or sofa will do – hold yourself with your palms face down outside your hips and body facing out.
2. Keeping your spine as upright as possible, draw away from the platform then bend your elbows to ninety degrees.
3. Squeeze your elbows towards each other as you extend your arms again.

Modification: Move your feet closer for more support, or further away to increase the challenge.

ELEVATED SIDE LUNGE

1. Standing with your right hip in line with the platform, allow your right foot to rest on the elevated surface and keep a soft bend in your left leg.
2. Keeping your left foot parallel and your hip, knee and foot stacked, lower your hip over your heel. You can drop as far as ninety degrees, or remain higher if you experience any pelvic discomfort.
3. Push through your heel to return to standing, squeezing the glute of the standing leg. Complete all your reps on one side before switching to the other.

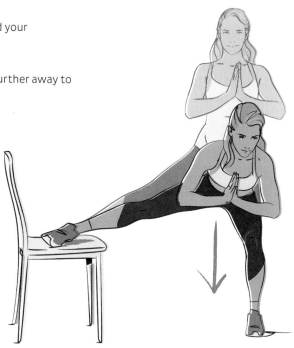

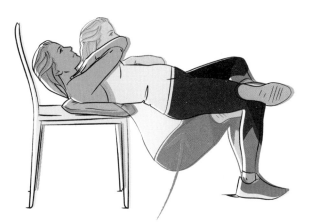

ELEVATED FIGURE-FOUR BRIDGE

1. Rest your mid-back on the platform, using a cushion for comfort, and cross your left ankle over your right knee. Pivot on your mid-back and lower your hips while actively opening the left knee to the side.
2. Push through the right heel and squeeze the glutes to draw your hips in line with your heart. Hold for a moment at the top and repeat all your reps on this side before switching to the other.

SEATED KICKBACKS

1. With your right leg folded in front of you, as in the pigeon position, allow your left knee to bend and rest comfortably to the side. Support yourself gently on your hands, resting them on the floor about 30cm (12in) in front of you.
2. Elevating your left knee, draw it slightly in front and then energetically behind you, squeezing the side of your left glute to get as much height and extension as possible.
3. Return to the start without lowering your knee back to the floor. Complete all your reps on one side before switching.

PLANK TO SIDE PLANK

1. From a high plank position, shift your weight onto your right hand and gently rotate your left shoulder as you reach your fingers to the sky. Exhale here, making sure the right elbow remains soft and you mindfully lift your right hip away from the earth.

2. Inhale to return through centre and repeat on the other side, counting both sides as one rep.

Modification: If you experience any discomfort in your wrists or lower back, try this on your forearms instead. For added support, allow your knees to touch the floor between side plank transitions.

DEAD BUG

1. Lying on your back, bring your knees to tabletop, with your shins parallel to the floor and your navel gently pulling in to maintain contact between your lower back and the floor. Float your arms in front of your chest.
2. As you exhale, simultaneously extend your right arm and left toe away, drawing your rib cage down to ensure you feel the work in your transverse abdominis rather than in your back.
3. Inhale through centre and switch sides. That's one rep.

Modification: Once you reach the five-month mark, modify by elevating your heart above your hips. Resting your shoulder blades on a wide yoga block or pillow should do the trick.

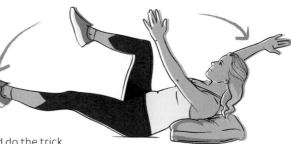

Balance the Bump

45 mins

Let's find your centre. Yes, it's ever-changing during pregnancy, but it's still there and there's ample to gain by honing in on it. This month's resistance workout helps you rehearse mid-line engagement, which grants you more control over every form of movement.

Start with the warm-up (page 78) and consult your level-specific instructions for the recommended weight, rep and set selection for each of the two circuits. As you'll have done plenty of unilateral movements, take note of how each side feels during the cool-down (page 80) stretches.

CIRCUIT ONE

KETTLEBELL CURTSY LUNGE CRUNCH

1. Hold a kettlebell in goblet position at your heart centre. Step back and across your standing leg into a curtsy lunge, wrapping your knee around the grounded ankle.
2. Push through the heel to stand, simultaneously bracing your core to bring your knee into a side crunch.
3. Tap your foot down to the floor between reps, or for an advanced progression try moving straight from crunch to curtsy.

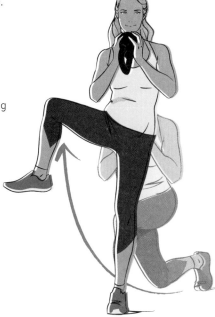

Mindful Mamas

Choose a light to medium weight that allows you to complete fifteen reps of each exercise in circuit one, focusing on the same leg with each consecutive move. Swap legs after each round, performing a total of four sets (two each side). For circuit two, perform the same number of reps, working both sides within the same set. Complete two sets.

Tandem Athletes

Choose a medium to heavy weight that allows you to complete ten reps of each exercise in circuit one, focusing on the same leg with each consecutive move. Complete three sets on one side, then three on the other (six total). For circuit two, perform the same number of reps, working both sides within the same set. Complete four sets.

Equipment

Medium kettlebell (6–10kg/13–22lb) or dumbbell

KETTLEBELL SINGLE-LEG DEADLIFT TO REVERSE LUNGE

1. With your weight in your right foot and a kettlebell or dumbbell in your left hand, hinge from the hip and lower the weight to shin-level.
2. Maintain a flat back and engaged core as you squeeze your right glute and hamstring to return to standing.
3. Upon standing, step back with your left leg and bend your knee into a reverse lunge. Push through the right heel to stand. That's one rep. Yep, the glute is meant to burn like that!

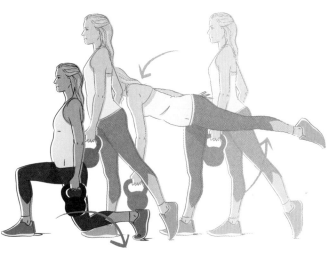

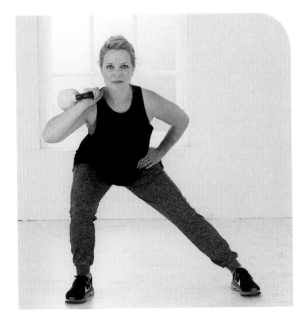

KETTLEBELL SIDE LUNGE

1. Stand in neutral position with a kettlebell in clean position by your shoulder, or alternatively use a dumbbell.
2. Take a big step out to the side, keeping the inner feet parallel and melting your hip over your heel.
3. Dynamically push off the floor and return to centre.

KETTLEBELL SWING

1. Assume a shoulder-width stance and hinge your hips as you drop the weight between your legs and dynamically squeeze your glutes as you swing through to chest or shoulder height.
2. Make sure you feel your glutes at the top of the movement; the dynamic squeeze will help to support the lumbar spine.

CIRCUIT TWO

KNEELING COUNTER PRESS

1. Come to a high kneeling position with one foot planted in front of you. Hold a dumbbell by the opposite shoulder – or progress to a kettlebell in clean position – and find a strong upright position through your torso.
2. Maintain this upright posture as you press the kettlebell or dumbbell straight overhead. Imagine your bum and belly button are working together – hips pressing forward and navel drawing in – to prevent collapse in the lower back.
3. You should feel this in the oblique and shoulder down the same side as the arm that's moving. Switch sides once you have completed all your reps.

DUMBBELL HIGH ROW TO ROTATION

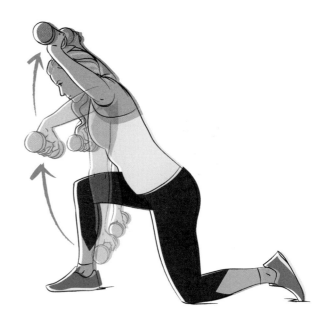

1. Stay in a split kneeling position, holding two dumbbells either side of the front leg, and lean forward through your torso.
2. Keep your core engaged and shoulders drawn together as you pull your elbows wide to frame your chest. At the top of the movement, pivot through your shoulders, keeping your elbows where they are, to rotate your palms facing up.
3. You'll strengthen the muscles supporting your shoulder blades as well as those injury-prone rotator cuffs.

BEAR PULL-THROUGHS

1. Come to all fours on your hands and knees, with a kettlebell placed just outside your left hand. Press through your toes and palms and hover your knees a few centimetres (an inch) off the ground, preventing any doming in your abdomen by tucking your hips and drawing in through the navel and rib cage.

2. Once you're stable in this 'bear' position, reach with your right hand to collect the kettlebell and pull it across so it rests just outside your right shoulder.

3. Reset your bear position, shift your weight into the right hand and pull the weight to the other side. That's one rep. Minimise movement in your knees and hips, resetting whenever necessary to maintain your form.

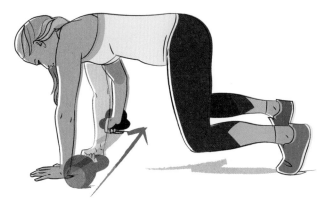

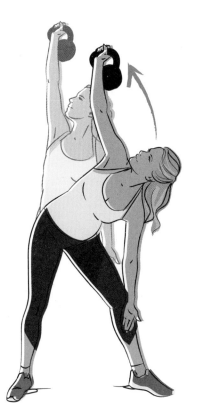

WINDMILLS

1. Stand with your feet just beyond hip-width apart, your spine in neutral, your left toe turned out to the side and a kettlebell or dumbbell pressed above your right shoulder.

2. Slowly slide the back of your left palm down your left thigh, maintaining a gentle bend through your left knee without turning the move into a mini lunge.

3. Squeeze your right oblique to return to standing, keeping your chest facing forward throughout. Switch sides once you've completed all your reps. You'll build stamina in your back and shoulder and strengthen the supporting muscles of your core and obliques.

Month Five Wellness Agenda

If baby's birth is the finish line in your nine-month ultra run, this month's halfway marker is a cue to slow down and take stock of how far you've come. In any endurance event, you have to make forward-thinking choices. Prenatal training is no exception, as your actions now could support you during delivery, aid postnatal recovery, enhance your energy levels as a new mum and accelerate your return to exercise.

- As you reduce impact activities, get creative and learn how to elevate your heart rate without defaulting to jumping and running. Try simple resources like gliders to maintain the pace and energy of your workouts – you can even continue doing burpees!

- Explore pregnancy-safe alternatives to supine exercises, such as bicycles and leg raises. Practise kneeling, standing and tabletop exercises that will keep both your core and your circulatory system in good working order.

- Use this crucial growth period as an opportunity to pre-empt and prevent lordosis – an exaggerated forward curving of your lumbar spine. Prioritise your posterior muscles with pulling movements and resistance-band work to improve postural strength and awareness.

- Continue working on your balance, but use more stable positions and variations as your growing bump makes offset exercises even more challenging. Split-stance deadlifts are a great example of a single-leg deadlift regression that will actually challenge your hamstrings more because you'll recruit the muscles more effectively when you're not wobbling about.

- Enjoy longer cool-downs when you can. Muscles in your chest, back and hips are likely to feel more constricted during high-growth periods. Taking the time to care for them now will improve their range of motion and your overall athletic performance in the late stages of pregnancy.

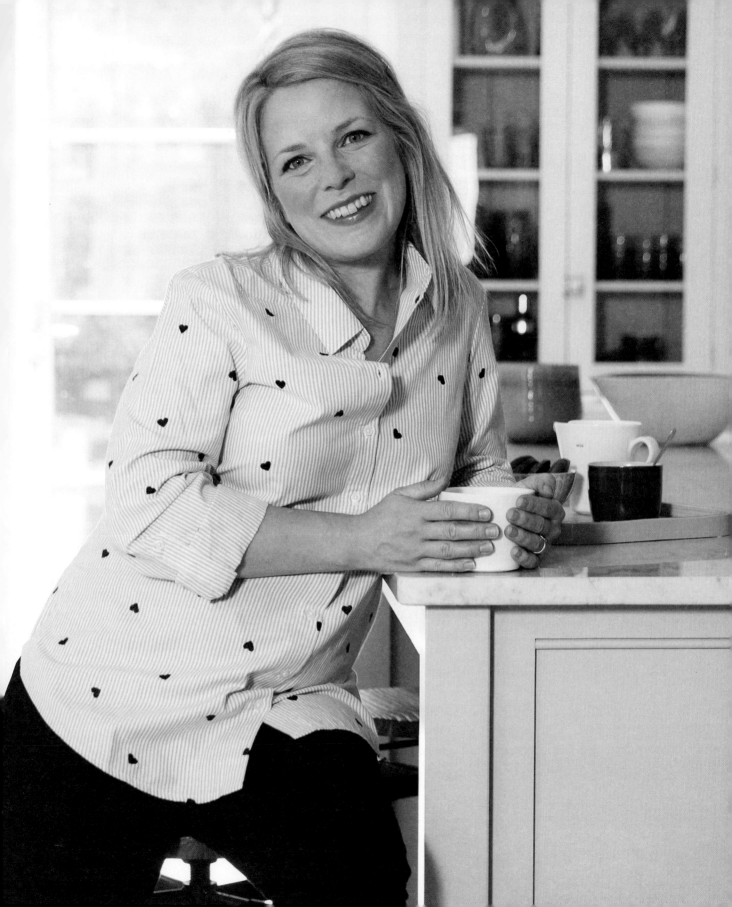

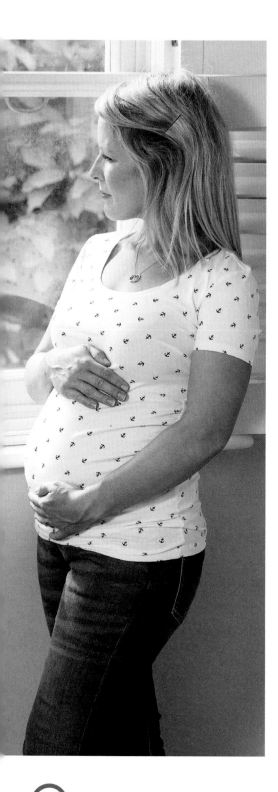

What is Happening to Your Body?

WHAT?

Month five typically ushers in a big growth spurt. Don't be alarmed if that's not the case for you – very strong abs may delay the visible growth spurt by another month or two. Whether your belly is blossoming or not, remember there is plenty of growth taking place beneath your bump. With that growth comes a dramatic increase in downward pressure on your pelvic floor, upward pressure on your diaphragm and even internal pressure on your inferior vena cava – the vein responsible for returning blood from your legs to your heart. Avoid lying on your back from this point onwards, as the supine position can further reduce circulation.

WHY?

Baby's body grows longer and plumper, and its spine becomes straighter, as it makes significant developmental leaps this month. That's why its residency in your womb is suddenly far more noticeable, and why you may feel reduced lung capacity as there is simply less space for your own organs. With all this growth dominant in the front of your body, it's natural for your spine to shift forwards gradually and weaken against the extra workload. Due to the combination of increased abdominal pressure and reduced spinal stability, it is wise to remove any running, bouncing or jumping from your exercise regime now.

SO WHAT?

The *MBB* workouts are low impact and have already been modified to help you work hard without compromising weakened muscles. It's time to put your foundational skills in pelvic floor breathing (see page 28) and deep-core activation to good use in order to prevent excess pressure in the abdomen.

There are still ample exercises that are beneficial as part of your training, and what you do now can play an important role in preventing or reducing the separation of connective tissue running down the midline of your abdominals. This condition – known as *diastasis recti* – can take months to rehabilitate postnatally; if returning to exercise after birth is a priority, then mindful exercise in the meantime is the most powerful resource in your maternal toolbox.

What is Happening to Your Baby?

BENEATH THE BUMP

Baby's growth is so substantial this month that size estimations transition from crown to rump to crown to heel. By the end of week twenty-one, your training buddy will weigh in around 360g (¾lb) and grow as long as an average carrot.

You'll have the opportunity to witness these changes at your twenty-week scan. While some expecting mums look forward to this scan – and to the optional gender reveal moment – others approach it with apprehension as baby is assessed for abnormalities. Talk to your partner or family if you are particularly worried, but know that the vast majority of scans reveal a healthy, thriving baby.

BUILDING AN ATHLETE

Your baby is already adept at protecting itself. This month it produces a lipid-based insulation called myelin, which cocoons baby's spinal cord to support communication between the brain and the nervous system. A two-part lining of soft, temperature-regulating hairs called lanugo plus a film of waxy, moisturising vernix forms all over baby's body, protecting it in the womb and preparing for an easier passage during delivery.

BABY PBs

Your increasingly active baby – who is enjoying flipping and turning in the womb while still having space to play – is already forming a unique identity. In fact, this month its fingerprints are fully formed. There is no one else in the world just like your baby. Now you can celebrate the halfway milestone and it won't be long before you make his or her very special acquaintance.

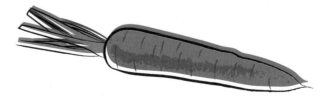

Fortify the Foundations

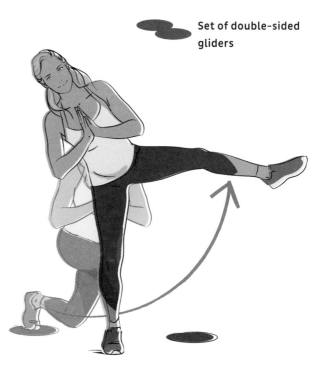

45 mins

It's time to step, rather than leap, into the second half of your pregnancy. Although high-impact exercise is inadvisable from this point, there are plenty of ways to get creative with your cardio. Gliders are a fun and effective way to maintain a heart-pumping pace that's kind to your joints and pelvic floor.

Find a hard-surfaced floor for this workout. After your warm-up (page 78), grab your gliders. Work through each exercise consecutively, using a timer to follow the work and rest intervals recommended in your chosen level. Rest for one to two minutes at the end of the circuit, then perform one more set for a thirty-minute workout or two more sets for a forty-five minute workout.

Mindful Mamas

Perform each exercise for forty-five seconds, resting for fifteen seconds before moving to the other side where relevant or moving on to the next exercise.

Tandem Athletes

Perform each exercise for sixty seconds, then move straight to the other side where relevant or move on to the next exercise.

GLIDER CURTSY KICK
---

1. With your left leg on the floor and your right foot on a glider, slide the right leg behind you into a curtsy lunge.
2. Press through the left heel to stand.
3. Once your feet are reunited, continue the movement of your right leg into lateral kick. Bend more deeply into your left leg to find balance. Only kick as high as you can without compromising stability. Switch sides after your chosen work interval.

Equipment

Set of double-sided gliders

BEAR DRAGS

1. Adopt a high plank position with your feet resting at hip width on gliders.
2. Maintaining a strong connection through your core and a sensation of lifting your shoulders away from the floor, pull each knee consecutively under your hips.
3. Hold briefly in this bear position, then reverse glide each foot back to plank. That's one rep.

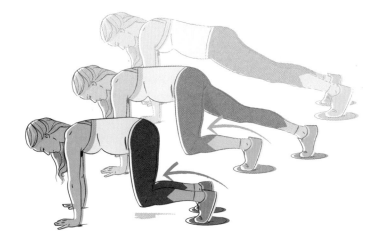

OBLIQUE GLIDE-UPS

1. Lie on your right side with your hips stacked and your right arm elongated so you can rest your head on your bicep. Your legs should be extended and your feet slightly in front of your hips so your body resembles the shape of a banana.
2. Rest your left hand on a glider by your shoulder. Simultaneously slide this hand towards your belly button while lifting your right side and left leg, gently squeezing your left waist. Switch sides after your chosen work interval.

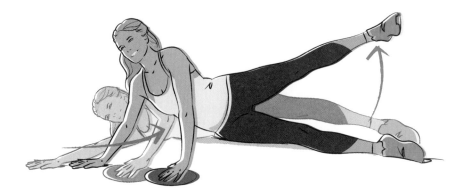

ROLLING PRESS-UP TO SINGLE-LEG PIKE

1. From a kneeling plank position, rest your right hand on a glider and your left foot on a glider.
2. Keep your hips tucked as you bend into your left elbow and slide the right hand away. You should feel your right lat and your full core working.
3. Return to centre, while wrapping your right foot across your left ankle and tucking your left toe into a full plank.
4. Now keep your hands static beneath your shoulders and glide your feet towards your navel as you lift your hips skywards.
5. As you return to full plank, lower your knees and resume your next rep. Regularly reset your abs to prevent doming. Switch sides after your chosen work interval.

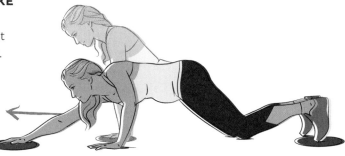

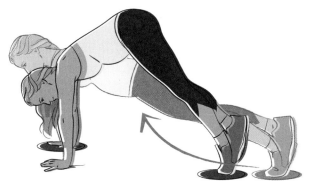

STATIC LUNGE REVERSE & LATERAL GLIDE

1. With your left leg on the floor and your right foot on a glider, slide the right leg behind you in a simple reverse lunge.
2. Return through centre, then slide the right foot out to the side as you lower your left hip over the heel.
3. Once again, your glutes should kick in quickly. Switch sides after your chosen work interval.

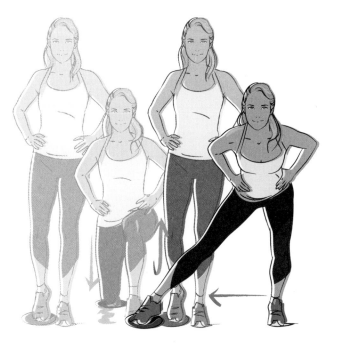

SUMO GLIDE

1. With both feet resting on the gliders, feet hip-width apart and toes in turnout, lower into a squat while sliding your right foot into a wide sumo position.
2. As you return to standing, draw the right foot back to hip-width distance, pulling through your inner thighs.
3. Repeat the above, this time to the other side. Both alternate sides make up one rep.

Modification: Take care on very slippy surfaces that you never lose control through your pelvis. You can modify with just one foot on a glider leading the movement for half the interval, before switching sides.

The Spine Aligner

45 mins

Don't be demotivated by the removal of core exercises performed on your back. Now is the time to master the ample challenging and effective alternatives available to you in tabletop, kneeling or standing positions, each bringing a multitude of benefits. Not only do these abdominal moves continue to galvanise your core, but they also work to stabilise the spine and prevent or reduce the lordotic (hollow back) posture that's so common in pregnancy.

After the warm-up (page 78), work through the four consecutive exercises of posterior-strengthening circuit one, then the four consecutive exercises of the band-resisted circuit two. Refer to your chosen level for your recommended reps and sets. Then lengthen the muscles you've strengthened with the cool-down (page 80).

Mindful Mamas

Choose a light to medium weight for circuit one. Three sets of fifteen reps should feel challenging but achievable. Follow with three ten-rep sets of circuit two.

Tandem Athletes

Choose a medium to heavy weight for the circuit one. Four sets of ten reps should feel challenging but achievable. Follow with three fifteen-rep sets of circuit two.

CIRCUIT ONE

WINDMILLS

1. Stand with your feet just beyond hip-width apart, your spine in neutral, your left toe turned out to the side and a kettlebell or dumbbell pressed above your right shoulder.
2. Slowly slide the back of your left palm down your left thigh, maintaining a gentle bend through your left knee without turning the move into a mini lunge.
3. Squeeze your right oblique to return to standing, keeping your chest facing forward throughout. Do all your reps on one side before switching.

SPLIT-STANCE DEADLIFT

1. This variation deadlift makes a comeback, having been introduced in month one (page 43). Adopt a strong and stable split stance.
2. Holding a kettlebell outside the thigh of your front leg, send your hips back and fold with a flat back until the kettlebell reaches your mid-shin.
3. Use the hamstring and glute of the front leg to pull yourself back to standing, realigning your pelvis under your rib cage at the top. Do all your reps on one side before switching.

Equipment

Medium kettlebell (6–10kg/13–22lb)

~~~ Resistance band

KETTLEBELL GOOD MORNING

1. Holding a kettlebell in goblet position by your chest – or, alternatively, squeezing the sides of a heavy dumbbell – softly bend through your knees and float your back to a flat position until your torso is just above ninety degrees to your legs.

2. Stop briefly here, connecting your core and drawing your shoulders back, before hinging from the lower back to return to your upright posture.

3. This movement should strengthen, but never strain, your lumbar spine. Look for a pull rather than a pinch in your lower back to ensure you're working with an appropriate weight.

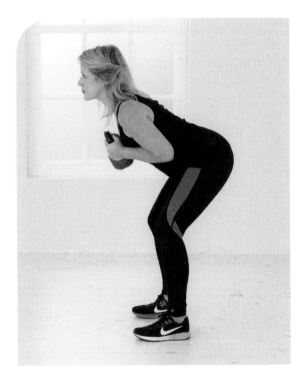

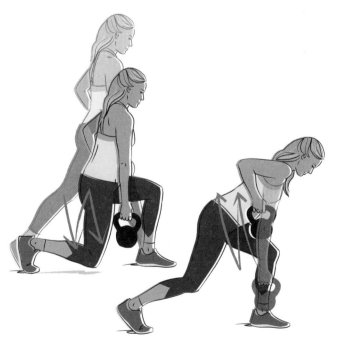

2 LUNGE 2 ROW

1. Hold a dumbbell or kettlebell in your right hand and ground down through your left leg. Step your right leg back into two deep lunges.

2. On the second lunge, hold the lowest phase of the movement and fold your torso over your left thigh. Now draw your elbow back in two complete rowing motions.

3. That's one rep. Do all your reps on one side before switching both arm and leg.

CIRCUIT TWO

BAND WALKS

1. Hold a resistance band by both ends and step down on the centre of it, your feet roughly hip-width apart.
2. Maintain a strong upright posture and work against the resistance of the band to take three lateral steps to the right.
3. Reverse the steps to your left. That's one rep. To rely on the strength of your glutes, keep your legs straight and avoid using momentum.

BANDED KICKBACKS

1. Come to all fours, holding the ends of the band under each palm and looping the centre around one of your feet.
2. Without rotating through the shoulders or hips, extend the banded leg until the length of your leg is level with your torso. Slowly bend your knee and return to a start position directly beneath your hip.
3. Complete all your reps on one side before switching. Continue resetting your navel and reinforcing a flat back position between every rep.

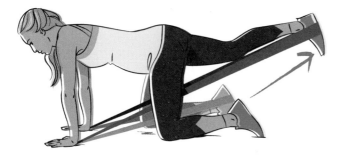

KNEELING SHOULDER OPENERS

1. Wrap a long resistance band around a pole, tree or banister (anything sturdy that won't topple over as you pull against it). Come to a high kneeling position with tension on the band as you hold either side of the band about 30cm (12in) in front of you.
2. Draw your navel in and, without moving your torso, exhale and pull the ends of the band to the sides of your hips.
3. Inhale and return, maintaining control against resistance. You should feel this in your lats and your core, plus you'll strengthen the stabilising ligaments of your hips and shoulders in the process.

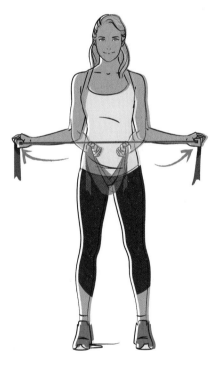

BANDED SERVING PLATTERS

1. Return to a standing position. With your palms turned up and about shoulder-width apart, hold the resistance band by your navel.
2. Keep your core engaged and your posture upright as you separate your hands. Your elbows should remain relatively static and tucked into your bump as you do so.
3. Slowly return to the centre, resisting the band as you do so. You're strengthening the small postural muscles of your shoulder blades, which should leave you feeling taller and more open through the chest.

Month Six Wellness Agenda

Your well-rehearsed, deep abdominal activation will be especially important this month as the core – along with the glutes – takes central stage. This month's workouts will give your body the complex postural support you'll need for the unique tasks of early parenthood: lifting and lowering baby in and out of the cot, manoeuvring the car seat, lifting and folding prams, nursing and holding baby on your hip while multitasking like only a mother knows how.

- Consider adding foam rolling to your warm-up. Myofascial release will help to ease constrictions in the muscle tissues and improve mobility during your workouts. This becomes especially relevant as supporting muscles compensate for your changing centre of gravity.

- As we incorporate upper-body isolating movements, support yourself on a Swiss ball or sofa to keep your heart over your hips. Engage your glutes and core so you don't dump into your lower back. This will help you learn to activate supporting muscles during the functional activities of early parenthood.

- Tune in to your alignment this month, as stacked or squared hips will help you fire the supporting muscles of your core and glutes far more effectively. Be aware of lazy positions and remain mentally present through every movement to make the most of your training time.

- Notice how effectively your heart rate soars during movements that simultaneously incorporate lower and upper body. Remain mindful of any breathing restrictions you have due to increased mucus production and take more rest if necessary after these exercises. These are now your safest and most effective form of cardio.

- If you do crave more intensive cardio, consider adding swimming to your repertoire. Even if you didn't enjoy pool time pre-pregnancy, consider that swimming offers a unique sense of weightlessness you'll appreciate now more than ever.

FOAM ROLLING FOR PREGNANCY

Using a foam roller can boost myofascial release, improving circulation to tight muscles and stimulating the Golgi tendon organ responsible for relaxing those muscles. The best time to foam roll is before a workout because it helps to improve your range of movement naturally and to promote safe and effective form. During pregnancy, the areas that tend to hold the most tension are the piriformis and iliotibial band (ITB; commonly the cause of sciatica), the lats and the thoracic spine. Here are three go-to foam rolling techniques to restore balance to the body:

1. Lean one hip – ideally between the iliac crest of your pelvis (the curved part at the top of the hip that sits close to the skin) and the peachy part of your bum – on the foam roller. Cross the same leg over the other knee to stetch the glute and intensify the massage. Use the grounded foot to push up and down gently as you roll to the top of your hip down to mid-thigh and back again. Stop and hold the roller if you feel any particular points of tension along the piriformis or ITB.

2. Elongate your lower arm and rest the side of your body – about 2cm (¾in) under your armpit – on the foam roller. Bend your top leg over the lower leg and push gently through the foot to move the roller down the side of your body.

3. Lie on your back with the foam roller just below your bra line. Avoid rolling below this point, but gently rock through your heels and lift your hips off the floor to glide the roller towards your shoulders and back again. It may also feel nice to leave the roller at your bra line and soften your head and shoulders to the floor.

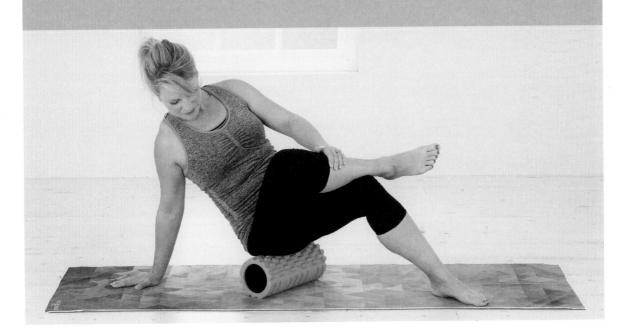

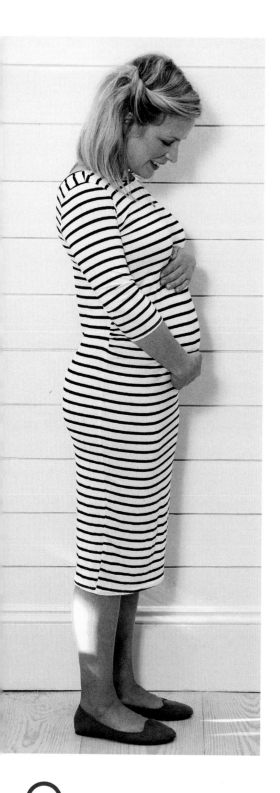

What is Happening to Your Body?

WHAT?

Bumping into fellow commuters? Overestimating the space between tables in a busy café? It can take a while for our brains to compute rapid changes to our bodies, and those pregnancy hormones can make the clumsy even clumsier. Besides any external changes, there are plenty of internal developments underway. Among the most notable is swelling due to fluid retention – particularly around the hands and feet – plus a pesky reservoir of mucus filling up your sinuses.

WHY?

Your increased blood volume causes extra fluid deposits around the body, on top of those from the mucus membranes. This extra fluid is useful to flush away toxins, but comes with some less welcome side effects such as swollen wrists and flu-like congestion. The swelling may put pressure on nerve pathways, which is the reason carpal tunnel syndrome is very common in pregnancy. Vary your hand position in plank and tabletop positions to reduce repetitive strain, and choose equipment with narrower handles for more comfortable workouts.

SO WHAT?

Avoid decongestants, as they work by restricting the blood vessels and could reduce nutrient flow to the baby. Try natural remedies instead: gentle steam treatments, hot lemon water and saline nasal sprays. If you feel as if it's harder to breathe, moderate your exercise so you have more time to rest, and remember to synchronise your movement with your breath so the working muscles get plenty of oxygen.

All this physical growth and extra fluid increases downwards pressure and may cause symphysis pubis dysfunction (SPD), also known as pelvic girdle pain (PGP). Symptoms include pain around the front of the pelvis. Exercise can help to reduce the symptoms, so try to keep moving, but prioritise pelvic floor and core strength to stabilise the area. Consider incorporating water-based exercise at this stage too; what feels like a 'wide load' on land feels a lot less cumbersome in the pool.

What is Happening to Your Baby?

BENEATH THE BUMP

As baby's previously polite pokes become more mischievous thumps, it may catch you off guard from time to time. Your baby's growth rockets this month, taking them to 36.5cm (14½in) long – a veg drawer equivalent to a head of cauliflower. He or she will be more active when you're at rest – often at nighttime.

Current belief is that baby begins experiencing rapid eye movement (REM) at this stage in its development, so if you do notice more sporadic twitches you may well be witness to new dream-induced activity. Baby can now distinguish sounds, including yours and your partner's voices, so feel free to start introducing favourite songs and lullabies. You'll be surprised by how comforting familiar sounds will be to your baby outside of the womb.

BUILDING AN ATHLETE

As your baby's head and body grow more proportionate this month, he or she will find a new ease of movement. Enjoy getting to know your budding gymnast. His or her eyelids will open this month as well; try stimulating sensory development by shining a torch on your bump.

BABY PBs

As well as gaining overall mobility, the tiny muscles in baby's face are growing stronger. Aided by its skin becoming smoother, it will be practising plenty of new facial expressions.

Facial expressions are useful for opening and closing the mouth to inhale and exhale amniotic fluid – a form of rehearsal for breathing. At twenty-four weeks, baby's lungs are developed enough that he or she could likely survive out of the womb with extra support from neonatal specialists.

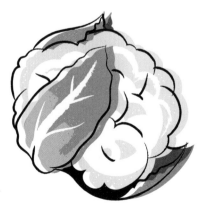

Growing Gains

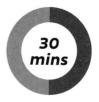

30 mins

After earlier high-energy workouts, enjoy pulling back the tempo and honing in on the core and the glutes with exercises that alternately target one then the other. Exercise variations that isolate one side of the body at a time will ensure you build symmetrical strength, which equates to a balanced, functional body.

Start, as always, with the warm-up (page 78). Then perform each exercise consecutively, performing both sides on exercises two, four and six, for sixty seconds each. Rest one minute, then return to the top and complete each move once again for forty-five seconds. Do one final circuit of thirty seconds work before giving your glutes a well-deserved stretch with the cool-down (page 80).

ARM WALK PLANK

1. Find your kneeling high plank position with your hips tucked, navel drawn in and hands directly below your shoulders. Retain a soft bend in your elbows.
2. Without changing your body angle, take four small alternating steps forward with your hands. You should feel a much deeper engagement in your core and side body.
3. Hold for a moment at the top, then reverse your steps.

Mindful Mamas

If you feel any strain on your lower back, try modifying your planks by placing your hands on an elevated platform. If you are experiencing carpal tunnel syndrome, use mini paralettes or sturdy dumbbells to maintain straight wrists.

Tandem Athletes

If the half plank (kneeling) variations feel very easy and you're confident that you're effectively containing abdominal pressure, try progressing to full plank (tiptoe) variations with the hands elevated or on the floor.

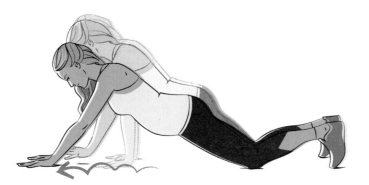

SEATED KICKBACKS

1. Bet you remember this one from month four! With your left leg folded in front of you, allow your right knee to bend and rest comfortably to the side.
2. Elevating your right knee, draw it slightly in front and then energetically behind you, squeezing the side of your right glute to get as much height and extension as possible.
3. Return to the start without lowering your knee back to the floor.

FEET WALK PLANK

1. Find your forearm plank, with your forearms parallel, palms down and a gentle curve in the upper back as you rise away from the ground.
2. Take four small alternating steps towards your navel with your toes, allowing your hips to rise skywards naturally. Continue elevating your shoulders away from the earth.
3. Hold for a moment at the top, then reverse your steps back to their starting position.

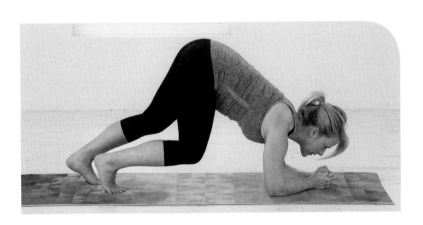

UPRIGHT CLAMSHELLS

1. With your right leg folded in front of you, allow your left knee to bend and rest comfortably behind your right foot.
2. Without momentum and without turning your left hip skywards, lift your left knee until you feel an intense squeeze in the top corner of your glute.
3. Hold for a moment before lowering to the start. Complete all your reps on one side before switching.

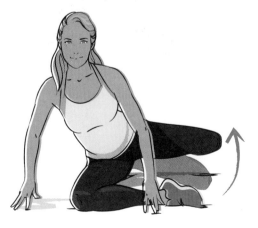

FLYING HALF PLANK

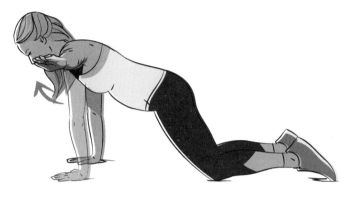

1. Find your kneeling high plank position once again. Keeping your hips and chest square to the floor, transfer your weight into your right hand and lift your left arm out to the side until it's in line with your left shoulder.
2. Hold for a moment at the top, feeling a squeeze between the shoulder blades and resisting any rotation through your midsection (which should still be engaged).
3. Slowly lower and alternate sides.

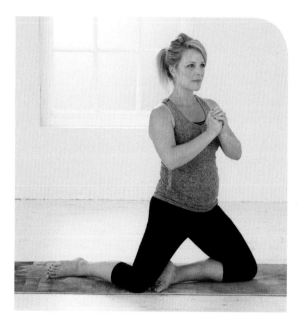

PIGEON BRIDGE

1. Enjoy revisiting this hip-stretching bridge variation from month three. Bring the working leg into pigeon position, folding the other leg behind you so your legs form a zigzag.
2. Squeezing your front glutes, lift your bum off your heels and dynamically push your hips up into a high kneeling position. Your back should form a straight line and your front hip should feel a stretch at the top.
3. Resist momentum and return slowly to the floor. Try to keep both hips pointing forward to make the most of this movement. The hip flexor will contract and lengthen, helping to counteract any overstretching that can take place as your bump pulls your hips forward.

YOGA FOR PREGNANCY

According to maternal health charity Tommy's, a single antenatal yoga class reduces stress-hormone levels by fourteen per cent and expecting mothers' feelings of anxiety by one-third. If you practise just one yoga position during your pregnancy, make it Malasana: the 'yogi squat'. It opens the hips, works as an active birthing position and is a great place to find stillness in mind and body.

Try holding for five breaths daily, counting in for five and out for seven. If symphysis pubis dysfunction (SPD) or muscle stiffness make this position uncomfortable, try a raised variation called Utkata Konasana with your heels wider and your hips above or in line with your knees. Little surprise it gives you more reign over your nerves – the translation from Sanskrit means 'Goddess Pose'.

When you need a less active practice, apply the same five breath cycles to a simple seated posture. Place one hand on your heart and one on your bump. Relax your tummy muscles and pelvic floor as you bring fresh air to your baby, then engage your pelvic floor and deep core to exhale up and out through the mouth.

Posterior Purpose

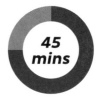

45 mins

A strong upper body will give you lifting, cuddling and nursing stamina as a new mum. If you do experience any symphysis pubis dysfunction (SPD, pain where the pubic bone meets the pelvis), big lower-body movements such as squats and lunges may begin to feel uncomfortable. Strengthening your upper body is a nice way to continue your training if the lower body needs a rest. In this workout we introduce some new movements and compound variations to work the total torso.

Remember to clock in to your workout with the warm-up (page 78). Work your way through each circuit one at a time. Refer to your chosen level for your recommended reps and sets. Focus on the bow and thoracic stretch in the cool-down (page 80); these target the supporting muscles of the lower and upper spine, which play a starring role in both circuits.

CIRCUIT ONE

SQUAT BICEP CURL

1. Stand with your feet hip-width apart, toes slightly turned out and your palms facing each other as you hold a dumbbell in each hand.
2. Lower into your squat and allow the dumbbells to drop towards the ground, but only go as low as feels comfortable.
3. As you return to standing, curl the dumbbells up to your shoulders, avoiding any swing in the elbows.

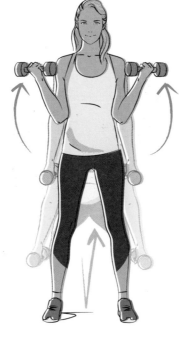

Mindful Mamas
Choose light weights to complete three fifteen-rep sets of circuit one. Then do a total of four sets of circuit two*, working one dominant leg each round and switching every set.

Tandem Athletes
Choose medium weights to complete three ten-rep sets of circuit one. Then do a total of six sets of circuit two*, working one dominant leg each round and only switching legs on the fourth set.

*The instructions for circuit two are specific to one working side only.

Equipment

Light to medium dumbbells (3–6kg/7–13lb)

Swiss ball

DEADLIFT TO LOW ROW

1. Maintain your foot position and neutral spine, but turn your palms to face you. Hinge from your hips with a soft bend in the knees to lower the dumbbells just below the knees.
2. Hold this deadlift position and draw the dumbbells in and back to frame your bump. Squeeze your shoulder blades then extend the arms once again.
3. After you've completed the row, push down through the ground and drive your hips into the dumbbells at the top of the movement. You should feel the work in your hamstrings and your bum.

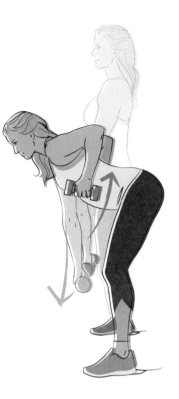

CHEST FLY

1. Resting your middle back on a bench, sofa or Swiss ball, hold two dumbbells with straight arms, maintaining a gentle bend in the elbows.
2. Keep your posterior chain engaged, drawing your navel to your spine and pushing your glutes forwards so you have constant tension through your torso.
3. Sweep your arms out to the sides and in line with your chest, then think about magnetically drawing the sides of the chest together as you return to centre.

TRICEP PRESS TO PULLOVER

1. Continue resting your middle back on a bench, sofa or Swiss ball and holding the dumbbells in front of you.
2. This time, draw your elbows down to frame your bump, magnetically wrapping the elbows around your spine.
3. As you extend the arms again, simultaneously reach them overhead so your elbows come to frame your ears.
4. Squeeze your lats and your chest to bring the weights back in line with your chest. That's one rep.

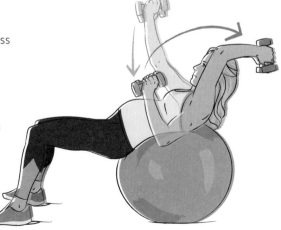

CIRCUIT TWO

DONKEY KICK

1. Come to all fours, placing one dumbbell in the nook of your left knee. Try to balance your weight equally down both sides of the body.
2. Squeeze your left glute to draw your knee to hip height. Maintain a slightly pointed toe and energetically contract your hamstring to hug the dumbbell.
3. Keep your hips and chest square to the floor throughout.

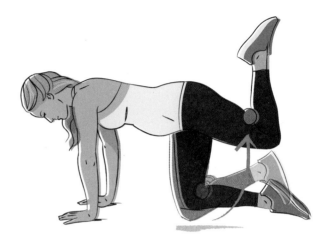

TORPEDOS

1. Lie on your right side with your right arm extended for a pillow and your hips stacked. Allow your left hand to rest lightly on the floor beside your chest for support.
2. Elevate your left leg about 30cm (12in) off the ground and flex both your heels.
3. Without rolling your hips, draw your right leg up to join the left. Hold for a moment, then lower the right only. That's one rep.
4. You are creating control and resilience in both the left oblique and the right inner thigh. For an extra challenge, hold a dumbbell against your left hip, increasing the load on the leg and destabilising the core by removing the supporting hand.

STAND-UPS

1. Kneel on your left leg and plant your right foot ninety degrees in front, holding the dumbbells by your sides.
2. Come to standing by pushing through your right heel, ensuring the knee tracks over the toe without any internal rotation. Return to kneeling.

Modifications: For a more advanced version, bring the left knee to your navel as you stand and the top of the left foot down to descend. For more support, tap the toe on standing and kneel down with a tucked toe.

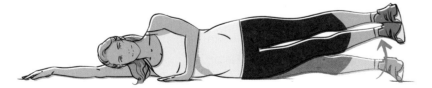

SINGLE-LEG DEADLIFT TO OVERHEAD PRESS

1. Standing on your left leg, with a gentle bend in the knee, hover your right foot and hinge from the hip to fold forwards until the dumbbells frame your mid-shin. Keep both hips square to the front or the floor.
2. Focus on the hamstring of the left leg to ascend. Simultaneously curl the dumbbells in and, once standing, press the dumbbells overhead.
3. Lower and uncurl the arms and repeat.

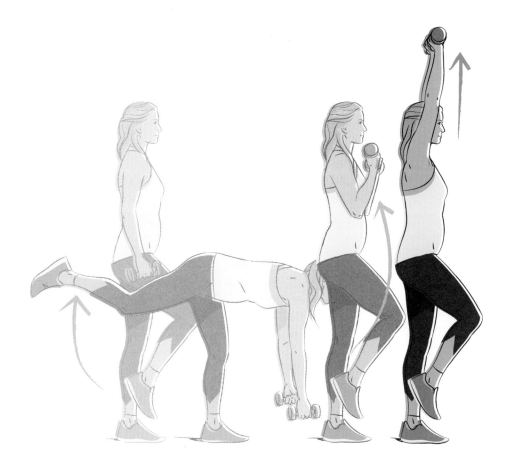

Maternal Mental Health

HOW TO TACKLE UNWANTED ADVICE

New research, changing practices and – let's be honest – general ignorance, can mean much of the advice we receive when pregnant is unhelpful or even upsetting. Try the following techniques to address unsolicited counsel or enlighten your enlighteners.

'THANKS' The most effective monosyllable to close any conversation before it begins.

SAY NOTHING, HEAR NOTHING Remember that information is ammunition to others, giving them an opportunity to weigh in on decisions you're busy weighing up. If there's something you'd like to consider without distracting contributions from others, keep the topic to yourself and you're less likely to invite unwelcome input.

USE THE GP GET-OUT CLAUSE Everyone trusts the authority of a doctor, so say you're following the advice of your GP.

BIRTH PREP FOR PARTNERS

Gone are the days when a dad waited in the pub for news of his baby's birth. Thankfully, partners play a far more active role in labour suites today. Birth preparation classes – which go by a variety of names including hypnobirthing, active birthing and yoga birthing – can offer valuable bonding time before baby's arrival, and help your partner feel less like a sitting duck and more like the rock by your side.

Classes are often run by doulas or qualified yoga-birth practitioners; the most popular ones fill up quickly, so consider booking ahead. A good workshop should cover the following:

- Partner massage and sacral pressure points
- Breathing to stimulate the body's natural pain-relief hormones
- Positions and movement patterns for an active labour
- Exposure to peaceful birth experiences
- How to write a birth plan midwives will actually read
- Mantras to support you through every stage of labour

TERIYAKI SALMON, CRISPY KALE & CHOI SUM

Serves Two

Omega-3-rich salmon promotes healthy skin cells. This recipe further enhances its superpowers by adding garlic, which acts as a protective antioxidant and provides lipoic acid, taurine and sulphur – all of which are essential for collagen production. A tasty antidote to stretch marks.

100g (3½oz) choi sum
100g (3½oz) kale
1 lime
1 red chilli
1 tbsp oil
2 spring onions
2 tbsp honey
2 tbsp tamari
2 x 150g (5½oz) salmon fillets (skin on)
4cm (1½in) fresh ginger
1 garlic clove
80g (3oz) quinoa

515 calories · 48g carbs · 21g fat · 39g protein

1. Preheat the oven to 180C / gas mark 4 and boil a kettle.
2. To make the teriyaki sauce: finely chop the chilli and peel and finely chop both the ginger and garlic. Mix in a bowl with the tamari, honey and half of the juice from the lime. Cut the choi sum stalks from the leaves. Cut the stalks into 1cm (½in) thick slices.
3. Rinse the quinoa and add to a saucepan with 300ml (1fl oz) boiling water. Simmer for 15 mins until cooked.
4. While the quinoa is cooking, heat 2 tsp oil in a medium-sized pan over a medium heat. Place the salmon in the pan skin side down and fry for 5 mins each side. Add the teriyaki sauce to the pan for 3 mins, then add the choi sum leaves and stalks and cook for a further 5 mins until the choi sum is tender and the salmon is cooked through.
5. Meanwhile, roughly chop the kale and place in a bowl with 1 tsp oil, spread out onto a baking tray and place in the oven for 5 mins until turning crispy and golden.
6. Thinly slice the spring onion into ribbons. Drain the quinoa and season with sea salt & black pepper. Stir in the remaining lime juice and the crispy kale.
7. To serve, spoon the crispy kale quinoa onto two warm plates, top with the choi sum and salmon. Drizzle over the remaining teriyaki sauce from the pan and top with the spring onion ribbons.

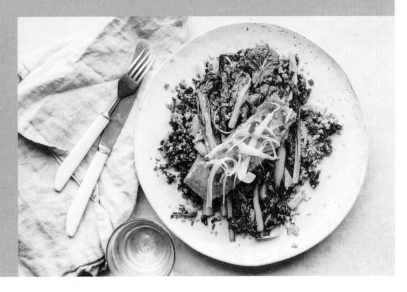

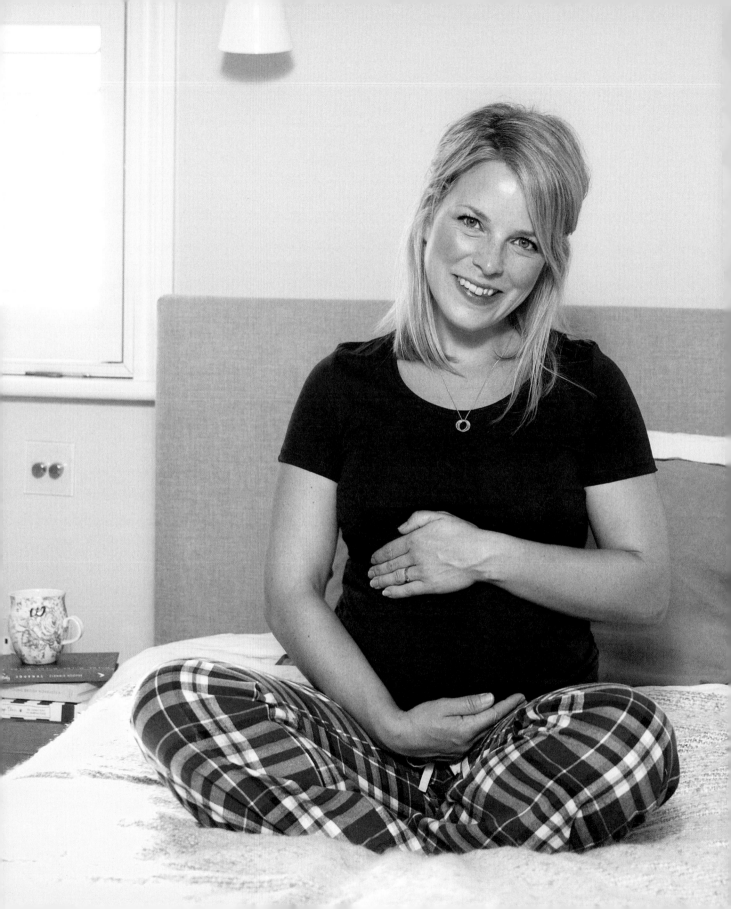

SLEEP BANKING

Speaking of annoying advice, perhaps the most common suggestion is to nap during the day. While it makes sense to bank more frequent sleep in anticipation of broken nights with a newborn, busy lifestyles don't often allow for leisurely daytime naps. Instead, focus on getting as much quality sleep at nighttime as possible, making extra provisions to keep comfortable and reduce bump-related disruptions.

INVEST IN A GOOD PREGNANCY PILLOW 'U'-shaped pillows cocoon you in the middle and keep you safely on your side so you don't wake panicking that you've rolled onto your back or tummy.

EAT LIGHTER AND EARLIER DINNERS Getting sufficient nutrition as your pregnancy progresses is essential, but with limited space for your dinner and less time to digest it in the evenings, frontload your calories and keep your last meal a little lighter to avoid sleep-depriving reflux or heartburn.

CLOCK YOUR HYDRATION While drinking ample water is your first priority, your second is to do the bulk of your hydrating before 8pm. This will ease the load off your bladder by bedtime.

WARM BATH, COOL ROOM While we often credit a warm bath or shower and a rise in body temperature with a quicker journey to dreamland, science shows it's actually the resulting drop in skin temperature after a bath that makes us feel drowsy. Maximise the contrast to reduce time spent counting sheep, keeping the room a cool 16–18°C (61–64.5°F).

MIND THE HEAD

Tension headaches remain common during pregnancy and are typically caused by dehydration, sleeplessness or anxiety*. Rather than tell you to drink often, sleep well and keep calm (and carry on), here's another useful tip to prevent headaches: max out on magnesium.

Magnesium is a mineral, stored in your bones and muscles, that plays a pivotal role regulating nerve and muscle function. Eating an insufficient amount is likely to make you feel fuzzy, weak and restless. Several studies link magnesium deficiency with chronic headaches, which is particularly relevant during pregnancy as both magnesium deficiency and persistent headaches can be symptomatic of pre-eclampsia. The good news is that there are lots of magnesium-rich foods at your fingertips. Incorporate a few servings from the following every day: spinach, swiss chard, dark chocolate, pumpkin seeds, avocado , black beans, tofu and bananas.

*If you suffer persistent and regular headaches during pregnancy, always consult your GP or midwife.

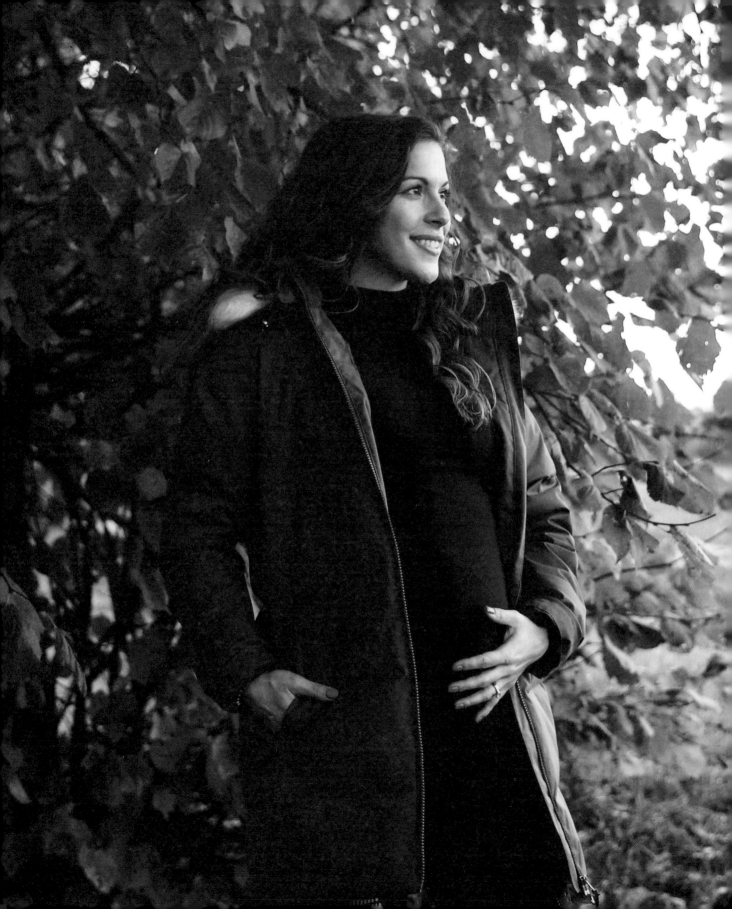

THIRD TRIMESTER

28–40 WEEKS

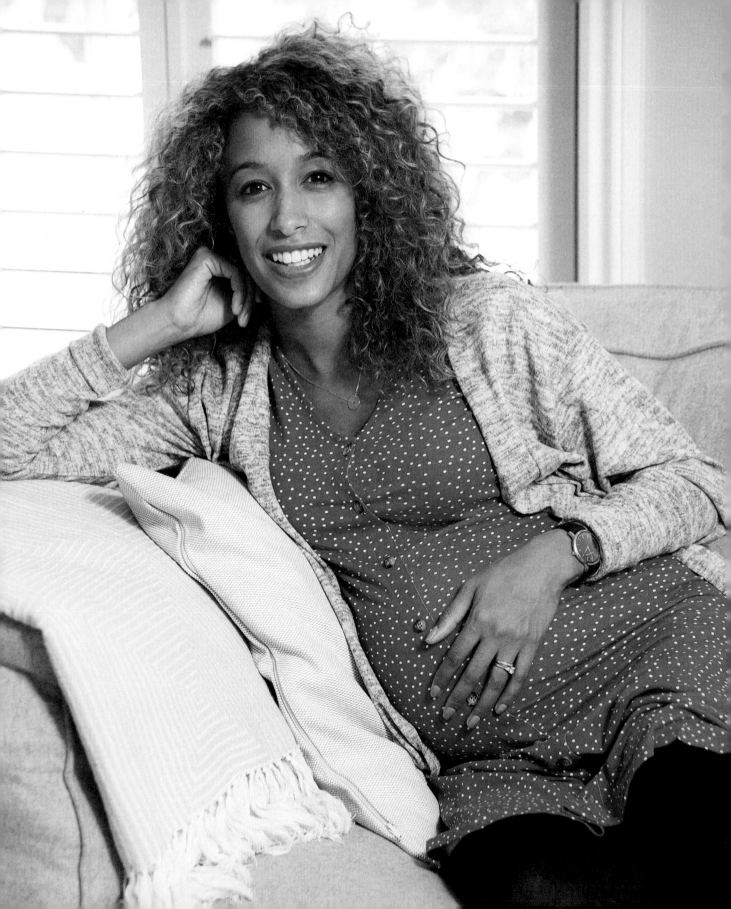

The Victory March

If we compare your pregnancy to an endurance event, transitioning into the third trimester is the equivalent of turning a corner and seeing the finishers' flag for the very first time. Though this is an exciting time for expectant mums, the truth is, the last few months of pregnancy can be challenging. My aim is to help you feel confident in yourself, prepare you for the challenges ahead and empower you to march through obstacles towards a podium finish like no other.

Physically, there is a huge amount happening to prepare your baby and your body for birth. We'll talk in detail about how to embrace the physicality of late pregnancy. But there is, perhaps, even more going on mentally. For me, pregnancy only felt real in the third trimester. Closing in on that finish line meant addressing anxiety over the birth, uncertainty about the ways in which having a baby would change my life (countless, but most of them brilliant) and frustration as fatigue slowed me down at work, in the gym and in my social life.

The good news is, the way you move your body plays a *huge* role in the way you feel as you approach your due date. While we reduce range and intensity of physical movement, we give new priority to self-awareness and that crucial mind-muscle connection. In this way, exercise becomes both a physical and psychological resource. This trimester's workouts provide the foundations for an empowered labour, plus highly specific physical preparation for life as a new mum.

Your Changing Body

The third trimester is all about standing to attention. Hopefully strangers show you everyday kindness by standing to offer you a seat. As important as it is to rest, incorporating regular movement into your days continues to be essential for your mental and physical well-being, and supports the incredible processes happening beneath your bump. Stand tall, devote mindful attention to both your body and your baby, and give yourself credit for how far you've come.

BRAIN

It's completely normal for you to experience anxiety or stress as you prepare for life with a baby. If panic strikes, tune into your breath (inhaling to a count of four and exhaling to a count of seven) to bring calm.

HEART

While your heart rate has stabilised, you may feel extra huffy as your bump snuggles up against your lungs. Adjust your exertion accordingly, moving slower or giving yourself more time to rest and re-oxygenate during workouts.

STOMACH

Your increasing appetite has only one way to go, and for good reason. As baby's weight can triple or even quadruple in the third trimester, you'll need to increase your calorie intake to fill up yours and baby's fuel stores. Current recommendations suggest an extra 300 calories; roughly an additional snack such as crudités and hummus, peanut butter on apple slices or yoghurt topped with granola.

BREASTS

Not only are your breasts still growing, but they're preparing to feed your baby. You may notice your nipples begin to leak a viscous, honey-like liquid – that's colostrum, a very nutrient-rich food on which your baby will thrive during his or her first few days.

OVARIES

The ovaries continue to work with the placenta to produce the hormones required for pregnancy. Oestrogen levels will begin to drop before birth, and much more dramatically after birth, in order to allow prolactin to stimulate milk production in the mammary glands. Mood fluctuations could be a sign of hormonal adjustments.

PLACENTA

As the weight of your baby dramatically increases, so too does pressure from your uterus onto other organs. It's important to minimise time on your back in order to aid blood flow to the placenta. If you have a low-lying placenta, take care to follow your physician's advice about exercise.

BLADDER

If you thought you had to pee a lot in your first trimester, prepare to put in the better part of a daily mile with even more trips to the loo. While the uterus moved up in the second trimester, it now takes up at least half of your abdomen and pelvis. If you do the maths, there simply isn't much space for your bladder.

BLOOD VESSELS

Regular exercise and position changes will boost your blood circulation to and around your increasingly squashed vitals. Varicose and spider veins become even more common in the third trimester. Both can eventually subside, but proactive prevention (remaining active) is your best chance to avoid them.

Beginnings & Endings

As you move through your third trimester, you'll encounter the most dramatic change in mobility. Some days you may feel you can take on the world (or a few heavy deadlifts, at least), but be prepared for less energetic days, too. Your third trimester warm-up and cool-down is designed to double as daily exercises when more energetic workouts feel out of reach. Simply repeat the warm-up for three to four rounds and give yourself permission to linger in your stretches, which become increasingly restorative the longer you spend in them.

THIRD TRIMESTER WARM-UP

Perform each of the following five exercises once through. Aim to spend roughly one minute on each, focusing on squaring your hips in order to effectively target your deep core and glutes and optimise pelvic stability.

x20

ALL-FOURS HIP LIFTS

1. Start in a neutral, all-fours position with a gentle bend in your elbows.
2. Minimising any rotation in your hips, draw a ski jump with your left knee, squeezing the side of your glute and wrapping your tummy muscles.
3. Replace the knee and do the same to the other side. Continue alternating through twenty reps, noticing if you gain any more mobility in the hip or feel more intensity in the glute as you work.

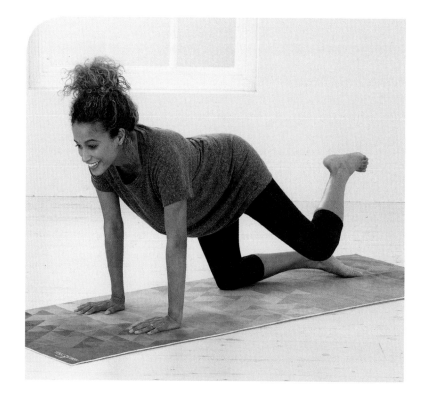

CAT-COW HOVERS

1. Come to all fours with your shoulders over your hands and your hips over your knees.
2. As you exhale, round your spine away from the floor and scoop your navel in. Practise gently lifting your pelvic floor as you do so.

3. From here, tuck your toes and hover your knees a few centimetres (an inch) off the floor for one full breath cycle. Think about wrapping your tummy muscles around your bump and squeezing the glutes, quads and inner thighs.

4. As you inhale, lower your knees and soften your spine down, shining your chest forwards and stretching through your lower back.

ALL-FOURS BANDED KICKBACKS

1. Remain on all fours, holding the ends of a resistance band under each palm and looping the centre around one foot.
2. Without rotating through the shoulders or hips, extend the banded leg until it is level with your torso.
3. Slowly bend your knee and return to a start position directly beneath your hip.
4. Complete all your reps on one side before switching. Continue resetting your navel and reinforcing a flat-back position between every rep.

Modification: You can do the same movement without the band. Focus on squeezing the glute and stretching through the back of the leg.

SQUAT TWISTS

1. From standing, hold your elbows in line with your shoulders, palms facing forwards.
2. Lower into a parallel squat, going only as deep as allows you to maintain working tension in your upper back.
3. Press through your heels to stand, simultaneously turning your chest to one side until you feel a gentle stretch in the middle back.
4. Return to a squat, alternating sides with each rep.

BANDED LATERAL STEPS

1. Assume a hip-width stance on a long resistance band, holding one end in each of your hands.
2. Keeping your spine in neutral, shoulders upright and your tummy muscles gently wrapping in, step one heel out to the side. Use a straight leg and fire from the glutes to do this.
3. Return through centre and alternate your reps.

THIRD TRIMESTER COOL-DOWN

Hold each of these stretches for at least as long as instructed. Use each inhale to find a little more length in your spine, and each exhale to gently soften into the stretch. You should see substantially, but comfortably, increased depth when you spend more than one minute in each position. If you have hypermobile joints, take care to avoid bouncing or overstretching.

BAND-ASSISTED SHOULDER STRETCH

1. Hold one end of a resistance band overhead, with your elbow bent until you feel a gentle stretch in your tricep.
2. Now reach behind your back to grab the band in the opposite hand.
3. Gently pull down on the band, intensifying the overhead stretch. Shine your chest forwards and continue drawing your shoulders together and tucking in your tailbone. Hold for at least fifteen seconds on one side before switching.

SPLIT-STANCE HAMSTRING & CALF STRETCH

1. From standing, split your stance forward and back and fold forwards with a flat back.
2. Firstly, bend into your back knee and kick your front hip back until you feel the length down the hamstring of the front leg. Hold for a breath.
3. Now bend into the front leg and lower your back heel until you feel the stretch down the calf of the back leg. Hold for one breath.
4. Repeat three to four times on one side before switching.

DIAMOND STRETCH

1. Take a seat on the floor or elevate yourself by sitting on a blanket or yoga block to relieve pelvic pressure. Bring the soles of your feet together to bring your legs into either a wide or narrow diamond.
2. Gently fold over your legs and use your elbows to help soften the knees to the side, stretching both the inner thighs and the hips.
3. Stay for as long as feels good, using your breath cycle to relax deeper into the stretch. Lengthen your spine on the inhale and fold deeper on the exhale.

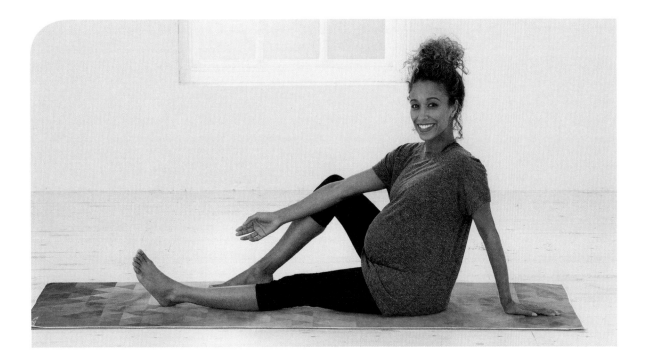

SIMPLE SEATED TWIST

1. Extend your left leg and bend your right knee, planting the foot roughly in line with your left knee. Sit tall through your spine and anchor your elbow inside the right knee.
2. Simultaneously pressing the right elbow out and the right knee in, gently turn your chest to the left. Keep the sit bones grounded.
3. Hold for a few breath cycles, then switch sides.

SUPPORTED PUPPY STRETCH

1. Rest your hands on a Swiss ball or elevated platform, shuffling your body back until your hips are square over your knees and your arms are straight.
2. Now allow your chest to soften towards the floor, feeling the stretch across your upper back.
3. This is a lovely stretch to hold through a few breath cycles, or to make more dynamic by rolling the spine away from the floor on the exhale and softening the chest towards the floor on the inhale.

UPRIGHT PIGEON STRETCH

1. Fold your right shin across your body and allow the left thigh to soften to the floor behind you.
2. Simultaneously soften into both hips, encouraging your right hip towards the floor and your left hip towards your right foot.
3. Keep your chest upright during this trimester. If you want a little more movement here, rise onto the fingertips and gently roll forward and back through your shoulders. Repeat on the other side.

Month Seven Wellness Agenda

The third trimester demands more rest for your body and more mindful awareness in movement. Still, exercise remains incredibly beneficial for your mind, your body and indeed your bump. It is far easier to prevent pregnancy-related pain or injury than it is to manage or treat it, and that's exactly what this month's workouts aim to achieve.

- Prioritise better form over bigger weights to maintain mobility as bump adds increasing load to the spine and pelvis.

- Continue foam rolling as per the second trimester (see page 107). If floor-based foam rolling becomes uncomfortable, try using a small massage ball on pressure points against the wall. Squatting as the massage ball rolls either side of your spine will help release tension in tight erector spinae (either side of the spine) muscles.

- Frequently stretch the back body to relieve any pressure on the sciatic nerve. Try to arc your spine gently in four directions: once in cat pose, once in cow pose and once to either side.

- Continue to strengthen supportive core muscles – predominately through compound (full-body) movements – to minimise the effects of lordosis (weakening of the lumbar spine).

- Remember that supine exercises (performed lying on your back) are best avoided at this stage. If you need to find your neutral spine, practise your pelvic tilts against a wall and find the natural midpoint with a soft curve in your spine.

- Take advantage of your relatively ample lung capacity by picking up the pace in this month's bodyweight workout. However, if you're feeling bunged up by extra mucus, build in longer rest periods between exercises and sets.

ACTION VS REACTION

Throughout the *MBB* workouts, we have been focusing on actively strengthening muscles that will support your changing body and maintain function of other muscles that can be compromised during this unique nine-month adventure. This approach allows you to optimise long-term physical fitness rather than focusing on short-term fixes to pregnancy-specific pain and/or injury.

However, the third trimester may require some additional support as your body adjusts to the increasing pressure of your rapidly growing baby. Below are some common problems you may face and how to adjust exercises mindfully to keep active safely and comfortably:

PELVIC PAIN Reduce range of motion during weightlifting.

BACK PAIN AND SCIATICA Use additional pre-workout foam rolling to release gluteal tension; stretch daily to restore spinal mobility.

HYPERMOBILE JOINTS Reduce range of motion to prevent overstretching the muscles and under-supporting the joints; avoid ballistic (bouncing) or active stretching in favour of passive or dynamic stretching.

OVERACTIVE HIP FLEXORS Incorporate daily hip flexor stretching – ideally for a minute or longer – plus foam rolling of any coinciding tightness in the piriformis of the outer hip, which can often overcompensate for tight or weak hip flexors.

REMEMBER TO LISTEN TO YOUR BODY If you feel any pain or discomfort while working out, ease off and adjust until you are comfortable. Always talk to your midwife or GP if you have any concerns.

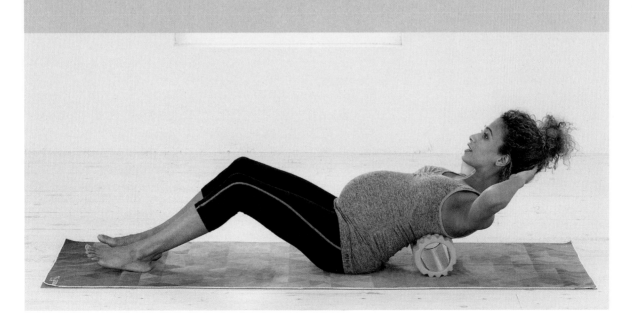

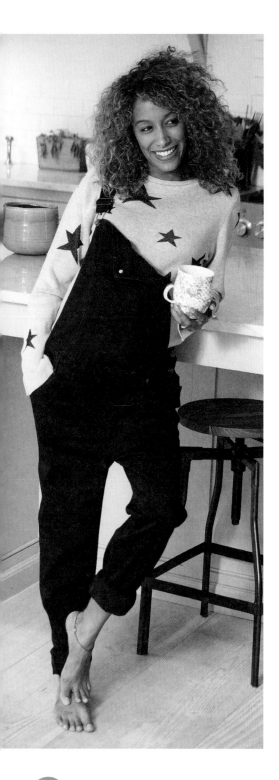

What is Happening to Your Body?

WHAT?

Prepare to get more acquainted with your uterus than you have with any organ before. There's a good chance it has now claimed dominant share of your abdomen and pelvis. Your first clue is your bladder, which has limited capacity and will be increasingly compromised over the next three months.

The good news: all that action on the inside means plenty of exciting action on the outside. Baby's movements will become far more definitive – maybe even visible. Try to look for patterns of movement rather than frequency, as this is what the doctors and midwives will ask you about during your antenatal appointments.

If you have any risk factors for developing gestational diabetes, you'll also be invited for a glucose screening test between twenty-four and twenty-eight weeks. It is a condition easily managed through diet and insulin injections but requires extra diligence before and after exercise. Do inform your care team about your training habits.

WHY?

Everyday movements turn your womb into a human rocking chair, sending baby to sleep while you're busy going about your day. Don't be surprised if he or she comes to life at night when you're beginning to slow down.

SO WHAT?

Your growing uterus will have some obvious side effects: you may feel more fatigue and require longer rest periods, while extra pressure on your sciatic nerve may cause some discomfort in the lumbar spine and down the backs of your legs. Stretching through the back body can help to relieve any sciatica (see cool-down, page 130).

Nerve pressure and reduced circulation can also cause leg cramps – particularly in your calves. Continue varying your body position and taking regular short walks to boost blood flow. If the cramps get very disruptive – especially at night – you could be a little low in electrolytes such as calcium and magnesium. Try naturally supplementing by including sources of both in your daily diet.

What is Happening to Your Baby?

BENEATH THE BUMP

While baby's growth rate is certainly on the rise, increased amniotic fluid is responsible for much of this month's uterine expansion. How much fluid you carry will have a significant impact on the shape and size of your bump. Having a very big bump does not necessarily mean you have a big baby.

You do, however, have a rapidly developing baby. Already he or she is beginning to shed the soft hair that grew in the second trimester. Baby's skin will also become plumper and smoother as it fills out to roughly the size of a coconut.

BUILDING AN ATHLETE

Towards the end of month seven, baby may start to move into a more active delivery position. By thirty-two weeks, many babies are already in a head-down position ready for birth; however, it can take up to thirty-six weeks for a baby to engage. You can use gravity to encourage this position naturally, with gentle inversions like down-dog.

BABY PBs

Baby may well be half his or her birth weight at this stage, growing to an average of 1.5kg (3.3lb). Every bit of growth in the womb now is preparing baby to thrive in the world outside.

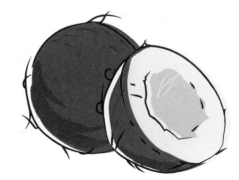

Lung Leverager

60 mins

This workout makes the most of your remaining lung capacity before further bump growth begins to make a serious dent on your diaphragm. Although we've cut out high-impact exercises, we're packing in plenty of compound movements that simultaneously challenge your lower and upper body. We also target similar muscle groups back to back, stimulating faster muscular fatigue and nudging your heart rate towards your fitness-maintaining anaerobic limit.

Prime your back, core and glutes for action with the third trimester warm-up (page 128). Circuit one targets the glutes, core and obliques through a playful 360-degree rotation. Work against the clock, using your chosen duration, with no rest. Things take a cardiovascular turn in circuit two. Work your chosen duration, but allow fifteen seconds rest between each exercise and each set.

Mindful Mamas

Work for intervals of 45 seconds in both circuits. Complete two sets per side (four full rotations) of circuit one and three sets of circuit two.

Tandem Athletes

Work for intervals of 60 seconds in both circuits. Complete two sets per side (four full rotations) of circuit one and four sets of circuit two.

CIRCUIT ONE

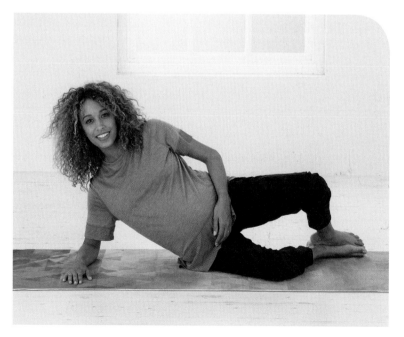

CLAMSHELLS

1. Lie on your right side with your knees bent and stacked so your heels are in line with your hips. Press through your elbow and actively draw the right side of your waist away from the floor.
2. Maintaining a strong line in your side body, draw your top knee open until you feel a squeeze in the side of your hip. Keep your hips square, so the movement comes from the glute rather than from the pelvis.

MERMAID LEG LIFTS

1. Come up on to your right hand, keeping your right knee grounded but extending your left leg long.
2. Flex the heel and lift the left leg in line with your hip. Control the movement from the glute, concentrating on squaring your hips, wrapping your tummy muscles and remaining open in your chest.

TABLETOP FIGURE-FOUR BRIDGE

1. Place your hands behind you with your fingertips pointing forwards. Cross your left ankle over your right knee.
2. Push through the right heel and squeeze the glute to draw your hips in line with your heart.
3. Hold for a moment at the top, then slowly lower to the floor.

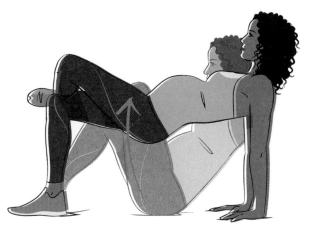

HALF PRESS-UP WITH OBLIQUE CRUNCH

1. Assume a half plank position. Do all your form checks – soft elbows, rounded shoulders, quads engaged.
2. Lower into a wide press-up, then lift your left knee and draw it out and up towards your left elbow.
3. Replace the knee in preparation for your next press-up. That's one rep.

SIDE-LYING TORPEDO

1. Turn to lie on your left side, with your left arm extended for a pillow and your hips stacked. Allow your right hand to rest lightly by your chest for support.
2. Elevate your right leg about 30cm (12in) off the ground and flex both your heels.
3. Without rolling your hips, draw your left leg up to join the right. You should feel this in the right side body. Hold for a moment, then lower the left leg only. That's one rep.

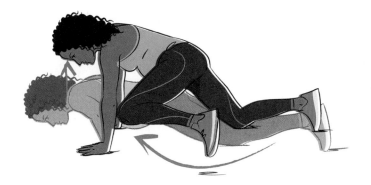

CIRCUIT TWO

OVERHEAD SQUAT

1. Stand with your feet hip-width apart and toes slightly turned out. Hold your arms overhead and draw your shoulders back and down.
2. Now drop your bum as low as you can without your chest rounding or heels lifting. This may not be very deep. That's OK – the priority here is to engage the back body. You should be able to lift your toes at the bottom, which is a sign your range is appropriate for your flexibility.
3. Inhale as you lower and exhale as you stand.

SQUAT HOLD CHEST PRESS

1. After you finish your last rep of the overhead squat, hold your lowest squat position. Bring your elbows in line with your shoulders, both palms facing forwards.
2. Simply draw your elbows together in front of your chest, stretching through your upper back, then draw them back in line with your shoulders and feel the stretch across your chest.
3. Don't let that upper body stretch fool you – that's just a lovely bonus on top of a *lot* of stamina-building in the legs.

HIP THRUST TO STANDING

1. Come to a kneeling position with your knees in line with your hips. Allow your bum to rest on your heels.
2. Squeezing your glutes, dynamically press up to a high kneeling position.
3. Keep your glutes engaged as you plant one foot and press through the heel to come to standing.
4. Reverse the movement, returning to kneeling then to resting on your heels. Alternate sides every rep.

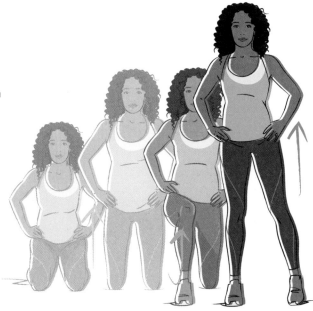

DOUBLE-PULSE LUNGE

1. Stand with your feet hip-width apart and your pelvis tucked under your rib cage.
2. Drive one leg back and lower into a lunge.
3. Before you return to standing, lift back to halfway and lower again until your knee hovers a few centimetres off the floor. Then drive through your front foot to return to standing.
4. Switch sides every rep. If you feel unsteady, use a chair, worktop or wall for support.

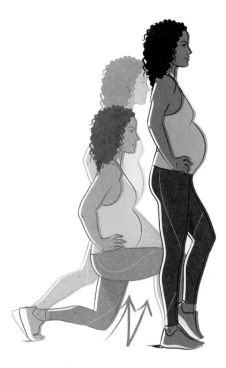

ALL-FOURS CURL AND HIP LIFT

1. Come to all fours, then extend your right leg as if performing bird dog without the arms.
2. Flexing the right heel, squeeze your knee to ninety degrees. Pause here and pulse the heel towards the ceiling. Resist losing tension in your middle to get extra height – small, controlled movements are superior to big, sloppy ones.
3. Extend the foot (don't lower the knee back to the floor) and complete a full set on one side. Switch after your chosen duration.

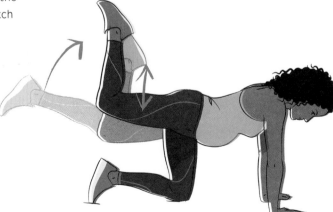

Two's Company

60 mins

Supersets train key muscle groups in a highly specific way. These eight exercises are paired to target the same or supporting muscle groups within each superset. That means the muscles reach sufficient fatigue to get a strength-boosting response, but the format also necessitates a period of rest between sets in order to optimise performance. Appreciate the value of rest in your workouts at this stage. Key muscles are already doing overtime and must be nurtured in order to effectively support you and your training.

Use the warm-up (page 128) to wake up all the muscles you need to support the following four supersets. Work through your chosen reps of each exercise, then rest for one minute after each superset. Prioritise the back body during your cool-down (page 130).

SUPERSET ONE

DEADLIFT TO CURTSY LUNGE

1. With your weight in your left foot, a kettlebell or dumbbell in your right hand, hinge from the hip and lower the weight to shin-level.
2. Maintain a flat back and engaged core as your squeeze your left glute and hamstring to return to standing.
3. Upon standing, step back and across with your right leg and bend your left knee into a curtsy lunge.
4. Push through the left heel to stand. That's one rep. Switch legs after you've done all your chosen reps.

Modification: If you feel unsteady, complete a traditional deadlift on two feet, before transitioning to your curtsy lunge.

Mindful Mamas
Choose a weight that feels challenging for twelve to fifteen reps of each exercise. Complete three rounds before moving on to the next superset.

Tandem Athletes
Choose a weight that feels challenging for eight to twelve reps of each exercise. Complete four rounds before moving on to the next superset.

Equipment

Heavy kettlebell (8–12kg/18–26lb)

Light to medium dumbbells (3–6kg/7–13lb)

Resistance band

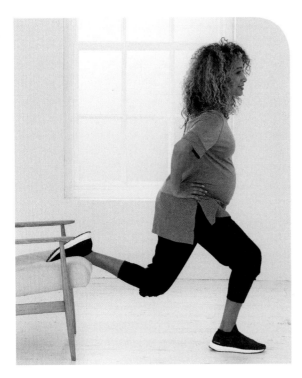

SUPPORTED SPLIT SQUAT

1. Rest the front of your left foot on a sofa, chair or alternative elevated platform. Ensure your right foot is distant enough that your knee tracks over your toe as you bend it.
2. Push your hips forward to encourage an upright position in your torso and lower your right hip as low as you can while remaining comfortable in the pelvis and steady through your middle.
3. Drive through your right heel to return to standing. Do all your reps on one side before switching.

Modifications: If you need extra stability, try holding a broomstick or similar in your left hand. If you feel any pelvic discomfort, reduce the elevation of your back leg and/or the range of your front leg.

SUPERSET TWO

VICTORY MARCH WALKING DEADLIFT

1. Holding dumbbells or kettlebells either side of your body, step one foot about 30cm (12in) in front of the other, draw your toes up and bend into the back leg as you fold gently, with a flat back, over the front leg.
2. Pause as the weights frame your knee, then pull through the hamstring to return to standing. Step the other foot through and repeat.
3. One rep includes both sides.

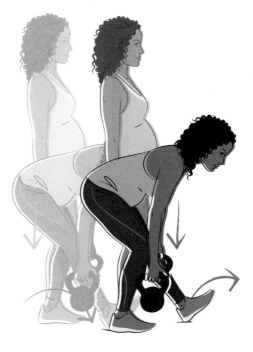

KETTLEBELL SWINGS

1. Hinge at the hips as the weight drops between your legs and dynamically squeeze your glutes as you swing through to chest or shoulder height.
2. Make sure you feel your glutes at the top of the movement; the dynamic squeeze will help to support the lumbar spine.

SUPERSET THREE

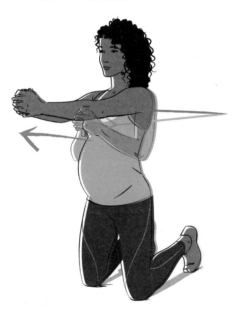

KNEELING BAND PALLOF PRESS

1. Anchor a resistance band and kneel with your left hip in line with the anchor. There should be enough tension in the band that you have to work to keep your hips square as you hold the band in both hands at your heart centre.
2. Without rotating through your hips (your left hip will want to draw back) extend your hands directly in front of your chest. Hold for a few seconds, then return to the start.
3. While this hits all your deep-core muscles, it also fires up the obliques of the side body closest to the anchor point. Do all your reps on one side before switching to the other.

KNEELING SHOULDER OPENERS

1. Wrap a long resistance band around a pole, tree or banister (anything sturdy that won't topple over as you pull against it). Come to a high kneeling position with tension on the band as you hold either end of it about 30cm (12in) in front of you.
2. Draw your navel in and, without moving your torso, exhale and pull the ends of the band to the sides of your hips.
3. Inhale and return, maintaining control against resistance. You should feel this in your lats and your core.

SUPERSET FOUR

DUMBBELL FLY TO CURL & PRESS

1. Holding a dumbbell in each hand, hinge from the hips and draw your arms out in line with your shoulders. Pause here, feeling the opening through your chest.
2. As you lower the weights, simultaneously come to standing. Then curl the dumbbells to your shoulders and press them overhead. Tuck your hips and gently wrap your abdominal muscles to support your lower back. That's one rep.

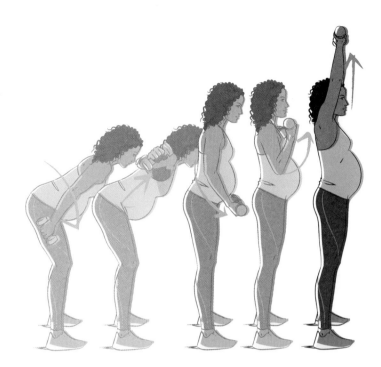

ALL-FOURS TRICEP KICKBACKS

1. Find a strong, comfortable all-fours position. Keeping a soft bend in the right elbow, hold a dumbbell in your left hand.
2. Engage your core to keep your chest and hips as square to the floor as possible, then lock your left elbow next to your midline and extend the arm o strengthen the tricep.
3. Do all your reps on one side before switching.

Modification: If you want an extra challenge, try extending your opposite leg as you perform the kickbacks.

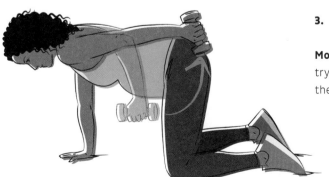

Month Eight Wellness Agenda

Typically the turning point in your pregnancy – when things begin to feel real and indeed your turning circle becomes rather larger – month eight provides a unique opportunity to own your march to victory. Staying mobile now is a game-changer for preventing awkward third trimester symptoms such as back and pelvic pain. Plus, it's the optimal time to break out the 'birthing ball', which has applications far more extensive than bouncing.

- Manage and reduce Braxton Hicks contractions by remaining well hydrated. If you do continue to drink caffeine, always pair your tea or coffee with a full glass of water.

- Allow more time to rest during and outside of your workouts.

- Aid and prevent sciatica with regular foam rolling, prioritising the glutes and piriformis by making a figure-four shape with your legs while massaging one side then the other.

- Try eating smaller, more frequent meals and snacks to prevent acid reflux during exercise and at night.

- As well as using the Swiss ball as a comfortable seating alternative (keeping your hips above your knees), explore new ways to incorporate it into your workouts. This month's weighted workout uses it in three ways: to strengthen muscles, to enhance joint stability and to provide additional spinal support.

- If you haven't started swimming, now is the time. If pool play isn't for you, there are plenty of modern benefits to garner from some old-school step aerobics! Establish three to four step patterns and do them each for one minute, repeating for as many rounds as necessary for your desired workout duration. This month's bodyweight workout will give you inspiration.

TRAINING WITH TWINS

While two babies doesn't exactly equate to twice the challenge, it is certainly true that certain symptoms of pregnancy will take effect sooner. Here's what you need to know about training with twins:

HORMONAL HIGHS Relaxin levels will be even more elevated, meaning joint instability and risk of injury are higher when carrying twins. Consider training with reduced load, and always be mindful of correct joint alignment during workouts.

BELLOWING BUMP As you would expect, your bump is going to be bigger with two babies – and it's going to get bigger faster. Your lungs will feel the squeeze, so you'll need to take longer rests more frequently.

CORE COMPROMISES As your belly stretches, so, too, do your core muscles. You are at greater risk of developing diastasis recti, so you may need to regress, or even skip, plank-based exercises in favour of compound movements that use the core for support rather than targeting it directly.

A FEAT FOR YOUR FEET With two pairs of feet in the womb, you'll want to keep two feet on the ground during third trimester workouts. Unilateral movements, such as lunges or single-leg deadlifts, will become particularly challenging on both the pelvis and the joints. Compensate by sticking with exercises that offer at least two contact points with the floor at any one time.

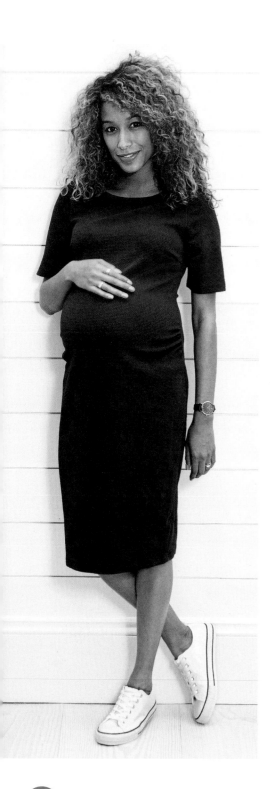

What is Happening to Your Body?

WHAT?

The end is in sight! It's worth bearing in mind that your due date is simply an estimation. Full gestation can vary according to a number of factors. Whether your baby arrives early, on time or has you dancing around your house in an attempt to induce an overdue delivery, by now your body is clearly preparing for his or her arrival. Intense pelvic pressure is probably morphing your walk into a waddle, Braxton Hicks contractions may have you wondering whether the real thing is just around the corner, and you may find your nipples begin to leak colostrum.

WHY?

Some women are more aware of Braxton Hicks – practice contractions of the womb that do not dilate the cervix or induce labour – and they're more common after your first pregnancy. Experiencing Braxton Hicks well ahead of your due date does not mean labour is imminent. Dehydration can make them more intense, so watch your hydration levels if you do find them frequent or uncomfortable.

Pressure against your digestive system makes it harder to process food. So while it is recommended that you increase your intake by a few hundred calories this trimester, you can probably only stomach small portions at a time.

SO WHAT?

While it's unlikely you'll deliver your baby this month, it's best to be prepared. Continue to train for physical strength and mental health, but also be sure to schedule rest and give your body time to recover between workouts. Aim to drink a full cup of water before, during and after workouts, to optimise your physical performance and mental awareness.

This little and often rule for hydration is just as relevant for nutrition, as smaller more frequent meals will reduce acid reflux symptoms. Eating smaller but more energy-dense meals (high in unrefined carbs, protein and healthy fats) two to three hours before working out will give your body sufficient time to turn food into fuel.

What is Happening to Your Baby?

BENEATH THE BUMP

With a fully developed brain and nervous system, the foundations of an independent immune system, and a digestive system that's primed for milk consumption, your baby is biding his or her time in the very cosy home you've created. By the end of this month he or she should move into an engaged position. If baby is determined to remain upright, your midwives and doctors will probably discuss techniques to help encourage it into a better position: acupuncture or a manual manipulation called an external cephalic version (ECV) are available options.

Babes in womb put on an average of 28g (1oz) a day at this stage – growing to an average of 2.5kg (5lb) and the length of a romaine lettuce leaf – so room for movement is fast disappearing. If you have any scans between now and delivery, baby's legs will most likely be in fetal position. While the volume of amniotic fluid will peak by thirty-six weeks, it will gradually decrease for the remainder of your pregnancy.

BUILDING AN ATHLETE

Although baby's skull remains soft and pliable – the plates will slide over each other during birth and the meeting points (fontanelles) will remain soft until up to eighteen months – there is ample you can do to help protect baby's brain in the meantime. Researchers in the United Kingdom have established a clear link between expecting mothers with higher iodine intake and higher IQs in the resulting children between ages one and nine years old. The mineral is required to make thyroid hormones, but also plays a pivotal role in fetal and newborn neurodevelopment during gestation and nursing.

A good source of iodine is cows' milk, which provides two per cent concentration of iodine. The researchers established that milk alternatives do not offer an adequate substitute, so if you can't drink dairy you may consider alternative sources such as seaweed, egg yolk and shellfish (remember it must be thoroughly cooked). Most pre- and postnatal vitamins also include iodine. The World Health Organisation suggests an RDA of 250mcg for pregnant and nursing mothers.

BABY PBs

Baby's cochlea – the part of the ear that communicates to the brain – continues to mature this month. That means he or she is increasingly recognising sounds from outside the womb, such as your voice or the music you like to play. If it feels as if baby is already mastering those drumming skills, you may have a mini musician in the making.

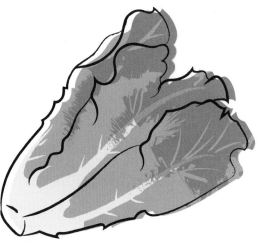

Two-Beats Cardio

Your pelvic floor is now getting enough of a workout by supporting the growing uterus, but your heart and lungs still need to be challenged in order to maintain optimum fitness. This workout uses low-impact movements to elevate your heart rate.

Following your warm-up (page 128), work through the three exercises of your pyramid, starting with twenty squat reps and reducing by two reps each round for a total of ten rounds. The duration of the monster walk and the bear crawl remain the same each set. Move on to the step circuit, working against the clock as per your level-specific instructions. If you like to match your movement to a beat, use a 120bpm playlist to work at a challenging, but achievable, pace. Warm? Don't forget your cool-down!

Mindful Mamas

Set the step on the lowest setting and do forty-five-second intervals with fifteen seconds of rest before the next exercise. Rest one minute and perform four rounds total, switching the leading leg each round.

Tandem Athletes

Set the step to the highest setting you can comfortably achieve and do sixty-second intervals with no rest between exercises. Rest one minute and perform four rounds total, switching the leading leg each round.

Equipment

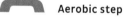 Aerobic step

PYRAMID CIRCUIT

SQUAT

1. Keep your feet hip-width apart and lower as far as you can, while maintaining good form and avoiding uncomfortable pelvic pressure. Do twenty reps.
2. These can be fast, but should never become uncontrolled. Go slowly enough that you stop at the bottom, rather than bouncing, and squeeze your way to standing, rather than jolting into your knees.
3. Once you've completed twenty reps, move on to your bear crawl. In the next round you'll complete eighteen reps, and so on, right down to two reps in the final round.

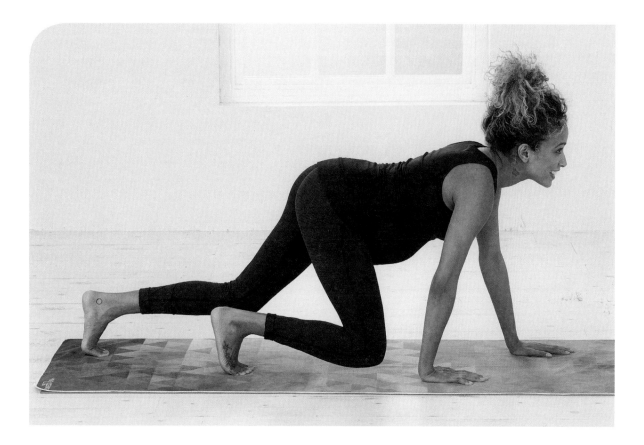

BEAR CRAWL

1. Come to all fours on your hands and knees. Press through your toes and palms and hover your knees a few centimetres (an inch) off the ground, engaging your tummy muscles to support your bump and gently tucking your tailbone to encourage a flat-back position.
2. Try to clear 3–4m (12ft) of space in front of you. Step forward with your left hand and right foot, then your right hand and left foot. Travel one full length forward, then reverse the movement back to the start. If you lose control of your core, or begin to feel this in your back, reset by lowering your knees before resuming.
3. One length forward and back equates to one round.

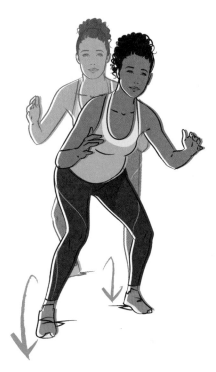

MONSTER WALK

1. Come to standing and lower into a squat position.
2. Holding this position, step your right foot forward, then your left to meet it. Now your left foot forward and then your right to meet it.
3. Repeat this 'squat walk' to the end of your designated space, then reverse the movement. Ensure there are no obstacles in your path as you reverse.
4. Performing one length forward and back equates to one round. Return to your squat.

STEP CIRCUIT

ECCENTRIC STEP-UPS

1. With both feet on the step, transfer your weight into your left leg and slowly lower your right foot to the floor. Avoid transferring your weight into your right foot.
2. Push through your left foot to return to standing, then transfer your weight over to the right leg and lower the left foot.
3. The slower you descend, the more strength you stand to gain in the working leg. Watch the knees to ensure they track over the toes throughout the movement, and to resist any internal rolling.

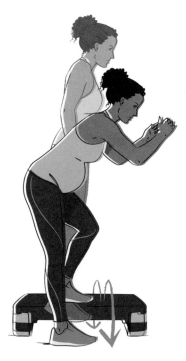

BOX STEPS

1. Standing in front of a stable step, march your right foot then your left foot onto the platform. Keep your knees gently bent and your core engaged.
2. Reverse your steps back to the floor. Then do the same on the left. Continue alternating with each step.
3. Move as quickly as you can without bouncing into your joints or stumbling over the step.

ELEVATED STEP CURL & LUNGE

1. From the floor, raise your right foot onto the step and pull your left heel into your bum.
2. Bring your left foot back to the floor and step the right leg back into a reverse lunge.
3. Step back through centre, then repeat to the other side, stepping up with the left and lunging back with the left.

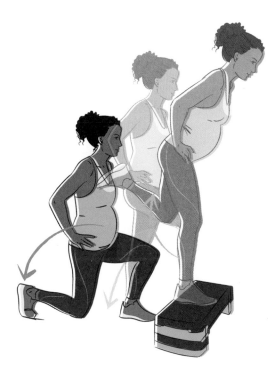

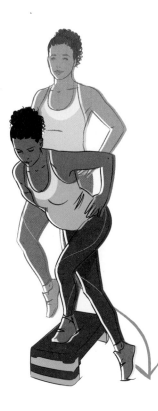

ECCENTRIC CURTSY STEPS

1. Stand on the step with your left foot slightly right of the centreline.
2. Float your right leg behind you and bend into your left knee to lower your toe to the floor on the left side of the step.
3. Squeeze your left quad and glute to stand. Maintain controlled movement, tapping rather than bouncing off the floor in order to protect the knees and optimise engagement through the glutes.
4. Perform a full set on one side before switching to the other side to complete the round.

Movers and Shapers

45–60 mins

Perhaps you've already begun sitting on a Swiss ball to relieve the load on your lumbar spine. Giving familiar routines a pregnancy-progressive upgrade, this workout will make you look rather differently at your comfy new 'seat'. Performed with and without weights, these Swiss ball exercises will strengthen key maternal muscles and help you adapt supine movements that are otherwise not recommended during pregnancy.

If you have any back or hip pain, add some foam rolling before the usual warm-up to release tension (page 107). Check your level-specific rep and set recommendations for both circuits. Rest between exercises and sets as required. Prioritise your hamstring, diamond and pigeon stretches in the cool-down (page 130).

CIRCUIT ONE

SWISS BALL SQUAT

1. With a Swiss ball between you and a wall, gently push your hips into the ball and use the extra support to encourage an upright position in your spine.
2. Bend into your knees and lower your hips, ensuring your feet are far enough away for the knees to track over the toes.
3. Pause for a second at the lowest point of your squat, then squeeze the glutes and press into the ball to stand.

Mindful Mamas

Do ten reps of the bodyweight exercises and choose a weight that feels challenging for fourteen to sixteen reps of the weighted exercises. Complete three rounds of each circuit.

Tandem Athletes

Do fifteen reps of the bodyweight exercises and choose a weight that feels challenging for ten to twelve reps of the weighted exercises. Complete four rounds of each circuit.

Equipment

 Swiss ball

 Medium to heavy kettlebell (8–12kg/18–26lb)

 Medium dumbbell (3–6kg/7–13lb)

SWISS BALL RAINBOW-SKATER STEPS

1. Standing naturally with a Swiss ball between your hands, take a wide step out to your right as you lower your left leg behind you into a skater position. Simultaneously circle the ball overhead to your right, so you finish slightly reaching out to your left.

2. Push through your right foot to stand, then take a big step to the left and reverse the circle with your arms. Both directions make up one rep.

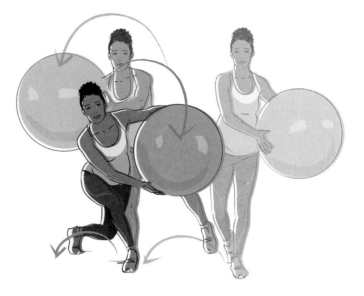

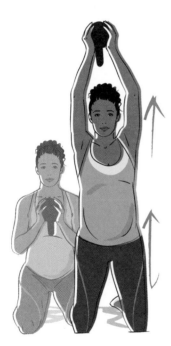

KNEELING HIP THRUST TO OVERHEAD PRESS

1. Come to a kneeling position with your knees in line with your hips. Allow your bum to rest on your heels. Hold a kettlebell or heavy dumbbell in your hands by your chest.

2. Squeezing your glutes, dynamically press up to a high kneeling position. Keep your glutes and core engaged as you press the weight directly overhead.

3. Reverse the arms, then reverse the lower body and slowly return to resting on your heels. That's one rep.

KETTLEBELL SWINGS

1. In a hip-width stance, hinge at the hips to let the kettlebell fall naturally between your legs, then push your hips forward, swinging the bell to shoulder level. Modify your kettlebell swings as required for your prenatal body. If you have less room to navigate your arms either side of your bump, reduce the travelling distance of the kettlebell and take shorter, sharper swings, focusing on the dynamic glute contraction at the top of the movement.

CIRCUIT TWO

SINGLE-ARM SWISS BALL CHEST PRESS
—

1. Resting your middle back on a Swiss ball, hold a medium to heavy dumbbell in one hand with your elbow wide and your palm facing forward.
2. Keep your posterior chain engaged, drawing your navel to your spine and pushing your glutes forwards so you have constant tension through your torso.
3. Rest one hand on your hip while pressing the weight from your shoulder to full extension. Switch sides after all your reps.

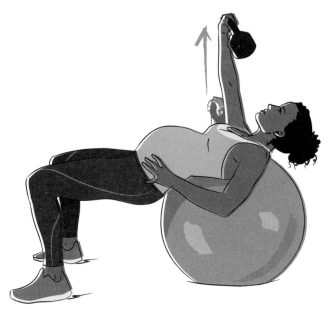

SWISS BALL ROLLOUT
—

1. Kneel down in front of the Swiss ball, ensuring you have sufficient padding for your knees. Rest your fingertips on the ball and lean forwards with your hips tucked and navel drawn in.
2. Maintain this position as you roll your arms out in front of you, naturally allowing your forearms to come to rest on the ball. Ensure your hips follow your arms and remain tucked, rather than sticking back behind you.
3. Pause while extended, then exhale to reverse the rollout and back to your fingertips.

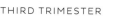

DUMBBELL ARCHER FLY

1. Come to a neutral standing position with two light to medium dumbbells by your sides.
2. Hinge slightly forward from the hips, ensuring your core remains gently engaged and your back supported in a straight line.
3. Simultaneously draw your right elbow wide into a high row and your left arm out to shoulder level with a straight arm (like a back fly). At the top of the movement it should look a bit like you're stringing a bow.
4. Reverse the movement and alternate the bent versus straight arm. Both sides equate to one rep.

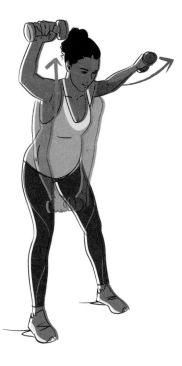

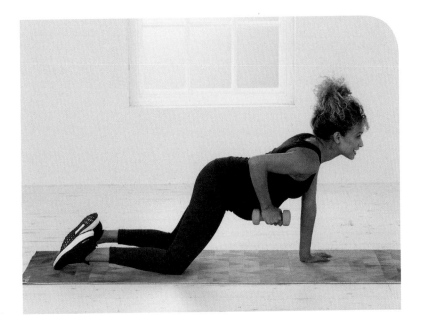

HALF-PLANK DUMBBELL ROW

1. In a high-plank position, hold a dumbbell in one hand and maintain a gentle bend in the elbow of the opposite arm.
2. Draw the first elbow straight back so it brushes your bump as you row the dumbbell, then slowly return to the floor.
3. Mindfully square the hips and wrap your navel or reset whenever you lose control from the midline. Do all your reps on one side before switching sides.

Month Nine Wellness Agenda

Welcome to a month of resting, nesting and personal besting. During the nine months of pregnancy, I acquired more respect for my body than I have at any other time of my life. Through your training over the last nine months, you've given your body all the tools it needs to move proudly and comfortably until labour begins, to support your body's instinctive efforts during labour, and to mend itself as you tend to your beautiful new baby. Let's finish as we began – with confidence, self-awareness and a sense of adventure.

- Rest and nest as much as required this month. If it becomes unrealistic to get to the gym or use equipment, prioritise the bodyweight workout as a whole or in parts.

- Continue to prioritise quality hydration and electrolyte intake.

- Structure your maternity leave to keep your mind busy, while permitting sufficient rest for your physical recovery. Make walking your primary daily exercise.

- If you enjoy your ongoing strength training, use kettlebell compounds (full-body exercises) to continue training your core safely.

- Continue foam rolling and stretching daily, particularly if you experience sciatica.

- Speak to your physician about baby's position and use active movement where appropriate to promote a head-down position for birth.

- Use free time to keep busy in the kitchen, preparing freezer-friendly meals that will nourish your body during postpartum recovery.

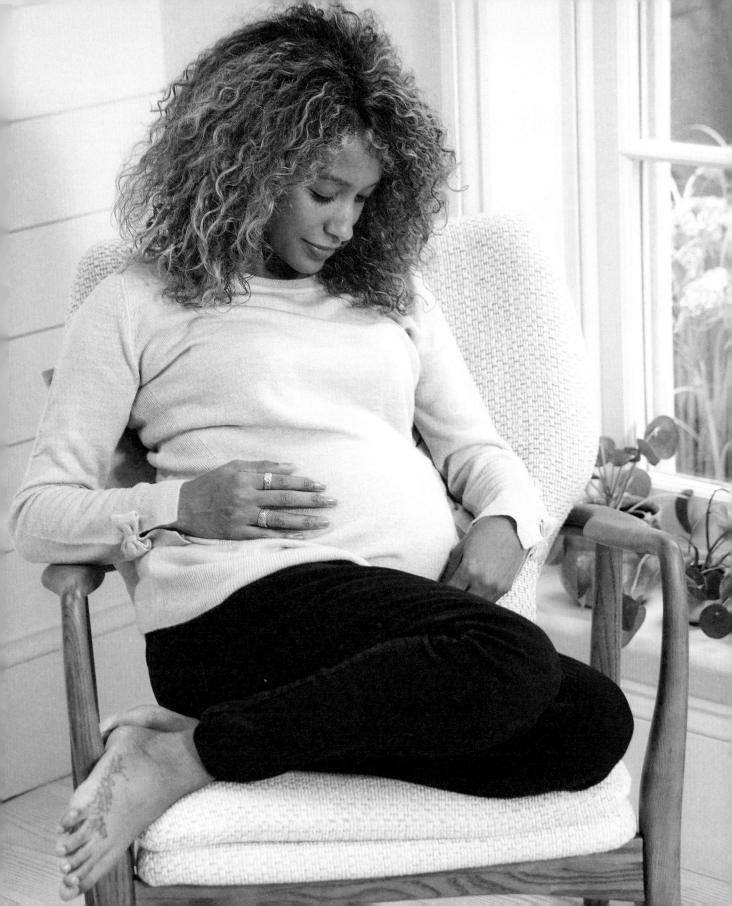

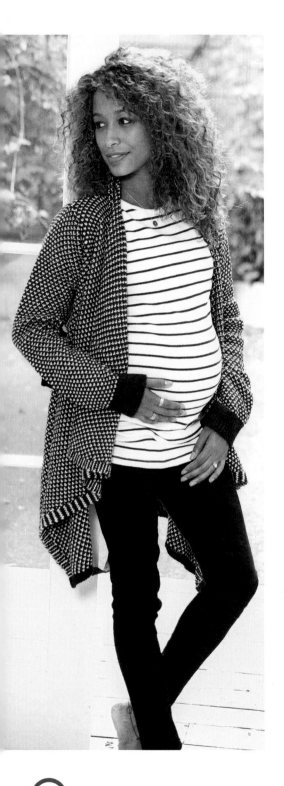

What is Happening to Your Body?

WHAT?

You'll reach full-term at thirty-seven weeks. Like any great victory, the real work is in the preparation. You've shown incredible commitment to a healthy and active pregnancy, and your body will thank you with the strength you need during and after your baby's delivery.

While you can certainly continue training in month nine, the priority now turns to rest. With time to spare, you'll naturally want to fill every waking second with productivity. Just remember that a nap can also be a productive use of your time.

WHY?

While some may tell you the nesting impulse – the urge to busy yourself around the household – is a sign of imminent labour, many mums also report that they nested feverishly for weeks on end until a forty-two-week induction. The more likely scenario is that your newfound energy has twofold origins: the visible descent of your bump as baby moves into an engaged position for birth, relieving your diaphragm and restoring your lung capacity; and the exhilerating reality that in a matter of weeks – maybe days – you'll be bringing a newborn into your home.

SO WHAT?

Nothing can come between a nesting expectant mother and her to-do list, so allocate non-negotiable time to rest. Book a pedicure. Swap a regular workout for a prenatal yoga class. Get hooked on a boxset and give yourself permission to binge watch for a whole day. Schedule naps. And by all means, pop these things on your to-do list so you can revel in the full gratification of crossing them out.

When you just can't slow down, devote your time to supporting your health and well-being as a new mum. Prepare and freeze lots of iron-packed meals to give you energy when you need it most. Draft an online shop, filled with easy healthy staples, so you can order in one click on your way home from the hospital. Stretch. Practise your birthing breaths. Do your kegel exercises – and remember to vary your position and movement, incorporating them on all fours, during squats and while you walk.

What is Happening to Your Baby?

BENEATH THE BUMP

Whether baby decides to hang tight until forty weeks or beyond, he or she is now ready to thrive in the world. Every day they continue to grow little by little. You may be nervously guessing his or her birth weight – your friends and family probably have stakes on it, too. During your next trip down the produce aisle, make way for the watermelon. That's the healthy size your little one will ripen to in the final weeks of pregnancy.

BUILDING AN ATHLETE

Go ahead and take that watermelon home with you. It's rich in arginine, which is an amino acid that helps to reduce blood pressure and aid circulation. It's also a refreshing snack to keep on hand during labour, keeping you hydrated and promoting the progress of your contractions.

BABY PBs

The average baby weighs 3.3kg (7.3lb) at birth – we can discuss in a few weeks' time whether that's a PB for you or the baby.

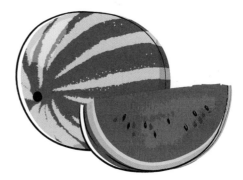

The Big Push

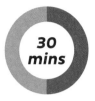

30 mins

Wordplay aside, there will be some days in month nine when you enjoy pushing yourself physically, and other days when a slower pace feels best. Listen to you body's cues. As we continue to focus on stability of the joints and balance from the core, always prioritise quality of movement over quantity of reps.

After your warm-up (page 128), and optional foam rolling, work through your recommended reps and sets of each workout segment. Feel free to use segments of this workout in isolation if shorter, more frequent exercise feels more manageable in the final weeks of pregnancy. Stretch daily, regardless of how long or intensely you've trained.

Mindful Mamas

Do eight reps of circuit one, switching legs after each set, for three rounds. Do eight to ten reps for three rounds of circuit two. Use stability-boosting modifications as required.

Tandem Athletes

Do ten reps of circuit one, working the same leg for each consecutive exercise before completing all three exercises on the other leg. Repeat for three rounds. Do twelve to fourteen reps for three rounds of circuit two.

CIRCUIT ONE

PISTOL SQUAT
—

1. Find a chair, bench or platform that is roughly level with your knees when you sit. Stand in front of it, balancing on the working leg while floating the other foot just off the floor.
2. Slowly drop your bum back and lower yourself to the chair.
3. Make sure your knee tracks over the toe. Without fully resting your bum on the bench, return to standing.

Modification: If you need extra support, try holding a broomstick or similar in the opposite hand to counterbalance.

PIGEON BRIDGE

1. Bring the working leg into pigeon position, folding the opposite leg behind you so your legs form a zigzag.
2. Squeezing the front glutes, lift your bum off your heels and dynamically push your hips up into a high kneeling position. Your back should form a straight line and the front hip should feel a stretch at the top.
3. Resist momentum and return slowly to the floor. If this movement becomes uncomfortable, place a yoga brick under your bum for extra support.

STEP-UP

1. Using a bench or platform that is ideally knee height or slightly higher, place one foot on the platform and drive through the foot to extend the leg.
2. Slowly lower down, without letting the knee roll in. Avoid using the other leg to help you lift away from the floor.

Modification: If you need extra support, try holding a broomstick or pressing against a wall with your opposite hand to counterbalance.

CIRCUIT TWO

RECLINE SHOULDER SQUEEZE & SWEEP

1. In a seated position with your knees gently bent in front of you, create a soft C curve with your spine as you roll your shoulders roughly forty-five degrees to the floor.
2. Holding this position, draw your elbows back in line with your shoulders and squeeze your upper back muscles.
3. Now draw your arms parallel again and keep them straight as you sweep your arms towards the sky. Hold for a moment at the top then return to the start. That's one rep.
4. If you lose control in your core or feel any lower-back discomfort, reset by sitting tall before continuing your reps.

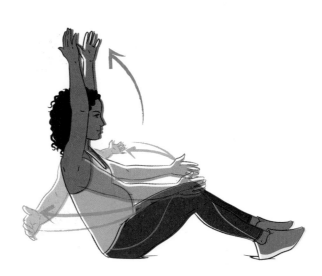

WIDE-LEG CHILD'S POSE TO PRESS-UP

1. Ensuring your knees are well cushioned, find a wide-leg child's pose with your knees roughly double hip-width apart. Allow your hips to melt between your heels as you release tension from your back and shoulders.
2. Transfer your weight forward onto your hands, checking there's a straight line from the back of your neck to the back of your knees. Tuck your hips and wrap your abdominals.
3. Maintaining tension in your core, lower your chest and bend your elbows to the sides. Exhale to return to extension and back into child's pose for as long as required between reps.

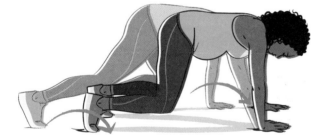

FOUR-WAY BEAR CRAWL

1. Find your bear hold and clear enough space to move about 30cm (12in) in any direction.
2. Place your right hand 30cm (12in) in front of you and step your left foot forwards.
3. Repeat with the left hand and right foot so you're square to the floor again. Now reverse back to the start.
4. Finally, step your right hand and right foot 10cm (4in) to your right, then follow suit with your left hand and left foot.
5. Reverse back to the start. One full movement forward and back, then side to side, counts as two reps.

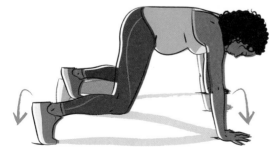

BREATHE EASY

These final few weeks are the perfect time to practise birth-specific breath control. There are several techniques out there – each designed to help you support your body during labour – and it's important that the techniques you choose feel natural and instinctive to you. These are the two that resonated most with me:

GOLDEN THREAD BREATHING A useful distraction during contractions, golden thread breathing is a simple visualisation strategy. As you inhale, visualise yourself drawing a long golden thread from the pit of your stomach. As you exhale, visualise that thread slowly fluttering through your lips. I paired this visual with a four-second inhale and seven-second exhale. The longest contractions are around sixty seconds long, so that's just five or six breaths until a rest.

CAFETIERE BREATHING You may never look at your morning brew in the same way again, but this technique for active labour proved extremely effective for me. As you inhale, imagine drawing the plunger up. As you exhale, send the breath downwards and imagine you're pressing the ground beans down. If you catch yourself breathing *out*, come back to your breath and focus on breathing *down*. Espresso, anyone?

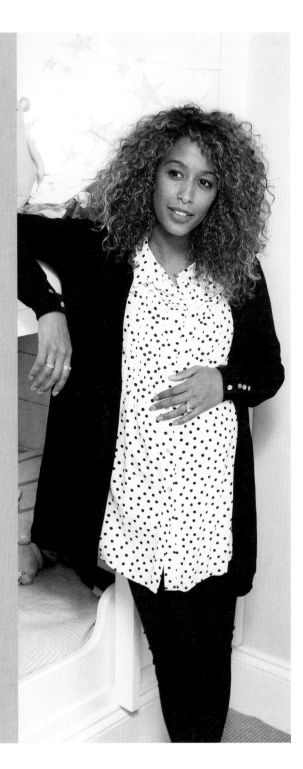

Power & Perseverance

40 mins

Beginning with compound movements that hit the biggest muscles, and finishing with a focus on smaller muscle groups, this workout is designed to be effective and challenging without causing muscular fatigue. Exercises have been selected to open the front body while strengthening the back body, which is helpful prep for the physical challenges of early motherhood.

Follow your warm-up (page 128), and optional foam rolling, with three rounds of both circuits, choosing an appropriate weight to feel achievable but challenging for your level-specific reps recommendation. As with your bodyweight workout, you can divide these circuits between two workouts. Your cool-down awaits (page 130).

CIRCUIT ONE

ECCENTRIC SQUAT TO SEATED

1. Find a chair, bench or platform that is roughly level with your knees when you sit. With your back to the chair, hold a large kettlebell in goblet position or medium dumbbells at your shoulders.
2. With parallel feet around hip-width apart or slightly wider, slowly lower your bum to the seat. Try to lower for a duration of five seconds or more.
3. Keep your weight in your heels as you return powerfully to standing.

KETTLEBELL CLEAN

1. Place a light to medium kettlebell in front of you and squat down to pick it up, palm facing you.
2. Pushing through your heels and bracing your core, powerfully trace the kettlebell up alongside your body, flicking your wrist at the top so the palm faces forward and the kettlebell rests on the back of your forearm at the top.
3. Reverse the movement and place the kettlebell back on the floor. That's one rep. Now do the same on the other side and continue alternating for your desired reps.

Mindful Mamas

Choose a medium weight to complete twelve to sixteen reps of the exercises in both circuits.

Tandem Athletes

Choose a medium to heavy weight to complete eight to twelve reps of the exercises in both circuits.

Equipment

 Medium kettlebell (6–10kg/13–22lb)

 Medium dumbbells (3–6kg/7–13lb)

LUNGE TO OVERHEAD PRESS

1. Holding the kettlebell in clean position by the left shoulder, find your neutral standing position with your hips gently tucked and your core engaged.
2. Now drop the right leg back into a reverse lunge as you simultaneously press the kettlebell up in line with your shoulder.

Modification: If you find this variation too unstable, take the left leg back instead so your right knee counterbalances your left hand. You can also use a wall for support, or press the weight at the top of the lunge instead of the bottom.

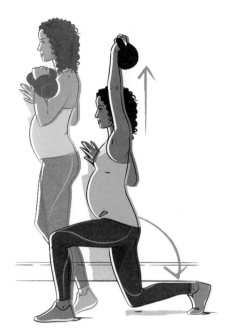

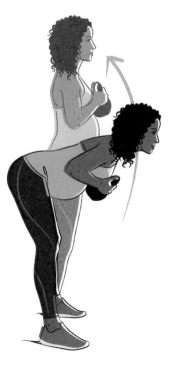

KETTLEBELL GOOD MORNING

1. Holding a kettlebell in goblet position by your chest, softly bend through your knees and float your back to a flat position until your torso is just above ninety degrees to your legs.
2. Stop briefly here, connecting your core and drawing your shoulders back, before hinging from the lower back to return to your upright posture.

CIRCUIT TWO

BALANCING BICEP CURL

1. Holding medium dumbbells at your sides, lift your left knee towards your navel and engage your core to find your balance.
2. Keep your elbows tucked into your sides as you curl the dumbbells towards your shoulders.
3. Slowly lower back to extension. Perform half your reps on one side, then swap the balancing leg for the remaining half.

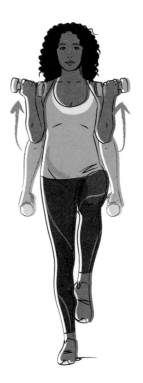

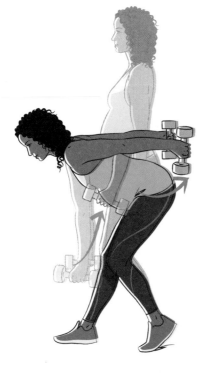

SPLIT DEADLIFT ROW TO TRI KICKBACK

1. Here we combine three movements to work both big and small muscles of the back body. Split your stance as per your usual split deadlift, holding dumbbells either side.
2. Lean forward into your deadlift, pausing as your hands frame your knees.
3. Hold this position as you row the dumbbells, then lock both elbows either side of bump and extend the hands into your tricep kickback.
4. Reverse the movement and return to standing. That's one rep. Perform half your reps on one side, then swap the dominant leg for the remaining half.

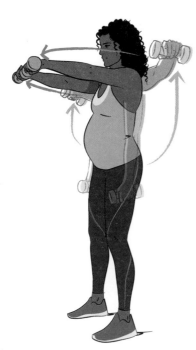

LAT FLY TO FRONT SWEEP

1. From a kneeling or standing neutral position, pull two dumbbells out to the sides, from hip level to shoulder level.
2. At the top of the fly, draw the dumbbells in to meet in front of your chest.
3. Reverse the movement in two steps. That's one rep. Check that you've fully returned to a neutral, engaged position between every rep. Avoid leaning forward through your hips or rounding forward through your shoulders.

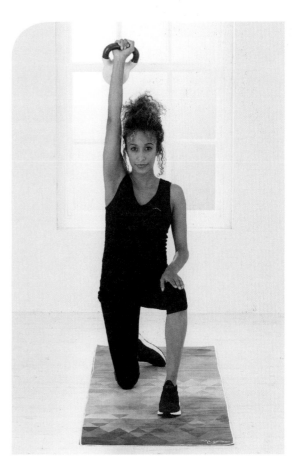

KNEELING COUNTER PRESS

1. Come to a kneeling position with one foot planted in front of you. Hold a dumbbell by the opposite shoulder – or progress to a kettlebell in clean position – and find a strong upright position through your torso.
2. Maintain this upright posture as you press kettlebell or dumbbell straight overhead. Imagine your bum and bellybutton are working together – hips pressing forward and navel drawing in – to prevent collapse in the lower back.
3. You should feel this down the oblique and shoulder on the same side as the arm that's moving. Switch sides after you've completed all your reps.

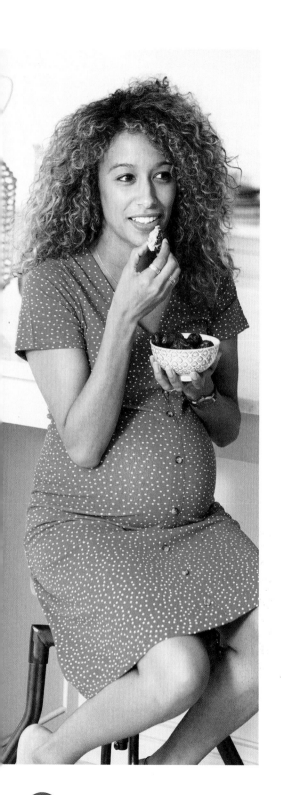

Finish Line Fuel

Here's your at-a-glance guide to bumping up the banquet for you and your near-full-term baby.

SWELL SNACKS

You may have expected your stomach to swell, but your feet? Oedema, or fluid retention, is common in late pregnancy, caused by a surplus of blood and fluid in the body. The good news is that your diet can help to deflate the problem.

GAGA FOR GARLIC Garlic is touted for its diuretic properties, which can boost kidney function and help to flush out excess water faster. More flavour, less inflammation.

POTASSIUM HAS PROMISE You have more fluid in your body, so you need more minerals to keep them chemically balanced. Top up on potassium-rich foods such as bananas, avocados and coconut water alongside ample water intake to maintain optimal hydration.

DE-PUFF WITH ANTIOXIDANTS Antioxidants, such as carotenoids and flavonoids, act to reduce oxidative stress and any resulting inflammation, de-puffing you from the inside out. These antioxidants give fruit and veg their bright colours, so eat the rainbow to boost the benefits.

MAKE A DATE WITH YOUR BABY

While curries have traditionally won all the credit for inducing labour, spicy food is more likely to cause one of the *signs* of labour rather than the event itself: diarrhoea. Dates, however, have had far more scientific success enticing babies to action. Researchers believe dates can simulate the effect of oxytocin in ripening the cervix and stimulating contractions. Studies have shown a link between 70g (2½oz) daily date intake in the lead-up to labour and a nineteen per cent increase in successful vaginal birth. Convinced? Here are three ways to dabble in dates . . .

STUFFED DATES Remove the pit and fill the date with nut butter or feta cheese. The fats and proteins in the filling will slow digestion of the dates' natural fructose, helping to stabilise your blood sugar, too.

DATE BALLS Blend the following in a food processor: 225g (8oz) dates with 70g (2½ oz) rolled oats, 3 tbsp nut butter or coconut oil, 1 tbsp cacao powder and 1 tbsp of chia seeds. Roll into fifteen bite-sized balls and store in the fridge for hungry (or impatient) snacking.

DATE TAGINES Take a leaf out of Middle Eastern cookbooks and include diced dates in your slow-cook stews or tagines (see page 171). They're traditionally paired with lamb or pigeon to complement meaty flavours.

SPICED STEAK FAJITA SALAD, PEPPERS & AVOCADO

Serves 2

200g (7oz) sweet potato,
skin on
1½ tbsp oil
1 tsp dried garlic
1 tsp ground cumin
1 tsp smoked paprika
2 x 150g (5oz) sirloin steak
1 roasted red pepper
1 avocado
1 lime
40g (1½oz) baby spinach
½ tsp red chilli flakes
(optional)
Sea salt and black pepper

559 calories · 39g carbs · 30g fat ·
38g protein

In the third trimester, baby absorbs 2mg of iron from you every day. The resulting store will sustain baby for the first six months of life. To boost its supply – and make sure you don't fall anaemic as a result – pair iron-rich foods (such as lean beef) with sources of vitamin C (such as red peppers), which aids iron absorption.

1. Chop the sweet potato into 1cm (½in) cubes and place in a medium saucepan. Cover with boiling water and add a pinch of sea salt. Simmer on a high heat for 10-15 mins until the sweet potato has softened.
2. Meanwhile, in a bowl, mix 1 tbsp oil with the dried garlic, half the ground cumin and half the smoked paprika. Season with a pinch of sea salt and black pepper. Rub the steaks with this.
3. Preheat a frying pan on a medium-high heat. Cook the steaks for 4-5 mins each side or until thoroughly cooked through. Remove the steaks from the heat and leave to rest for 5 minutes.
4. Thinly slice the roasted red pepper. Peel and de-stone the avocado; thinly slice.
5. To make the dressing, mix the remaining smoked paprika and ground cumin with ½ tbsp olive oil and the juice from the lime.
6. In a large bowl, toss the baby spinach with the sweet potato, avocado, roasted peppers and the dressing.
7. Thinly slice the rested steaks. Place the salad onto two plates and top with the steak. Sprinkle with chilli flakes, if desired.

LAMB SHOULDER TAGINE & BROCCOLI RICE

Serves 2

½ beef stock cube
1 brown onion
2 garlic cloves
1 sweet potato
40g (1½oz) dried dates
2 x 150g (5oz) lamb shoulder
2 tsp oil
1 tsp ground coriander
½ tsp ground cinnamon
1 tsp smoked paprika
200g (7oz) passata
20g (¾oz) flaked almonds
1 small head broccoli
Sea salt and black pepper

645 calories · 47g carbs · 28g fat ·
32g protein

1. Boil a kettle. Dissolve the ½ beef stock cube in a jug with 300ml (10½fl oz) boiling water.
2. Peel and finely dice the onion and peel and crush or finely chop the garlic. Peel and cut the sweet potato into 1cm (½in) cubes. Roughly chop the dates.
3. Season the lamb with sea salt and black pepper. Heat a medium saucepan with 2 tsp oil on a medium-high heat and cook the onion for 3 mins, then add the lamb to the pan and brown on all sides for 3–4 mins. Stir in the garlic, ground coriander, ground cinnamon and smoked paprika and cook for 1 minute. Then add the passata, beef stock, sweet potato and dates. Place a lid on the pan and simmer on a low-medium heat for 30 mins until the lamb is cooked through.
4. Meanwhile, heat a dry, medium-sized pan on a medium-high heat and toast the almonds for 2–3 mins until golden brown.
5. Grate the broccoli into a rice consistency using a grater. Heat the same pan you used for the almonds and add the broccoli rice with 2 tbsp water. Cook for 3–4 mins, stirring constantly until the broccoli has slightly softened.
6. Thinly slice the lamb shoulder. Spoon the broccoli rice onto two warm plates and top with the sauce and the lamb shoulder. Sprinkle with toasted flaked almonds.

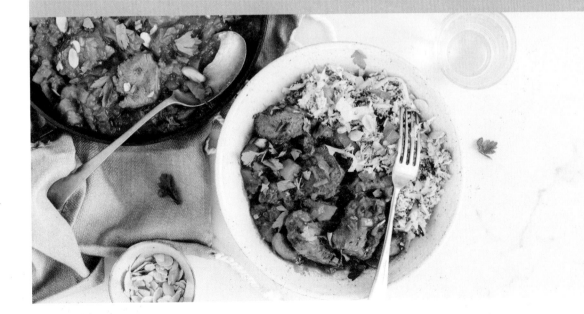

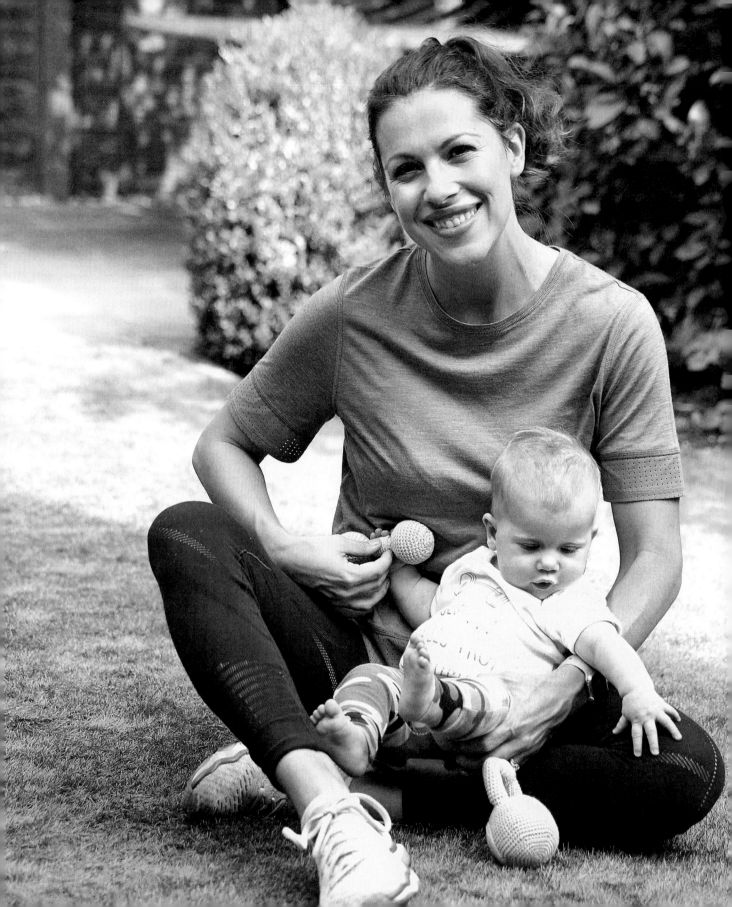

FOURTH TRIMESTER

0-12 WEEKS

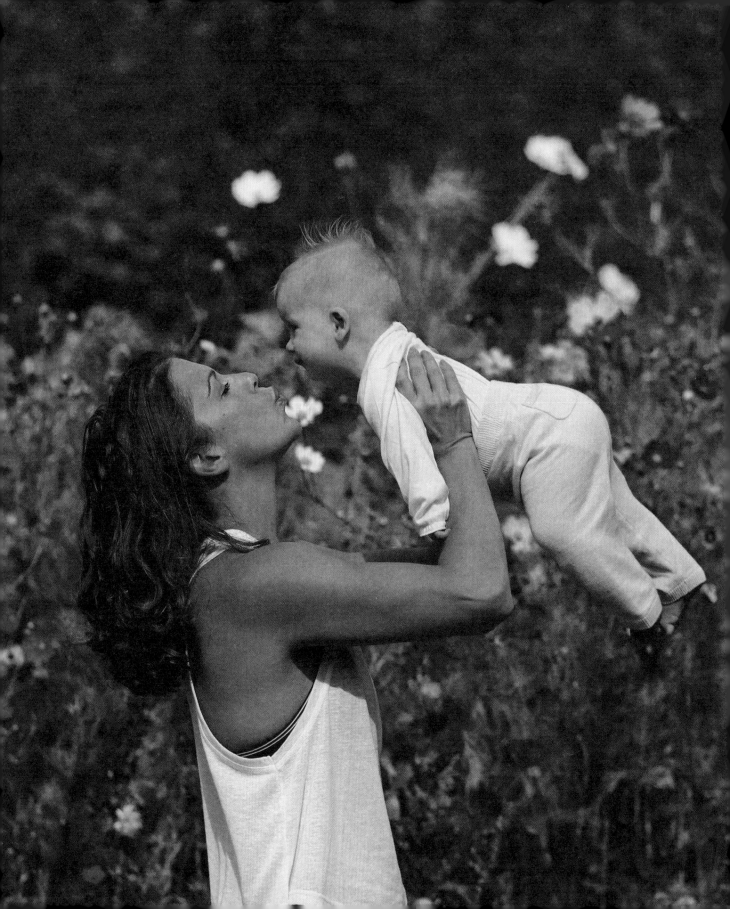

A Podium Finish

Congratulations, mama! Firstly, for finally meeting your baby athlete. Secondly, for arriving here on this page. If you have the time and energy to be thinking about exercise, you and your newborn are clearly thriving.

If exercise played an important role in your pregnancy, it's likely you'll be eager to return to structured movement. However, if you are here out of any sense of obligation, please know that there is no reward for returning to exercise before you feel ready. By training throughout your pregnancy, you have equipped your body with the tools it needs for optimal recovery from pregnancy and childbirth. Your return to exercise now should be a slow, steady and very happy journey.

The two workouts in this chapter are merely suggested movements to help you reconnect safely with your body. Between now and your six-week medical check-up – sometimes up to twelve weeks if you've had a caesarean – you will be doing well simply to get out of the house and push the pram most days of the week.

In recent years, a phrase has emerged to represent the first three months of early motherhood: the fourth trimester. I love this phrase because it serves as a reminder that, just like the three trimesters of pregnancy, everyone's postpartum recovery is unique. It also removes the pressure for new mums to do any kind of 'snapping' back into shape. You and your body have been through a lot. As you invest all your energy in nurturing your baby, sufficient self-love is essential to ensure you have enough left over for your growing family.

If you've had a terrible night's sleep, this 'self-love' may look more like a nap than a workout. However, if you are feeling energetic, it could involve a few restorative core exercises while baby plays on his or her mat, or some foundational squats and lunges while he or she enjoys the security of cosying up to you in a baby carrier.

There is no agenda this month, and therefore no Monthly Wellness Agenda in the subsequent pages. Now is the time to enjoy getting to know your baby, and to nurture the body that built him or her from scratch.

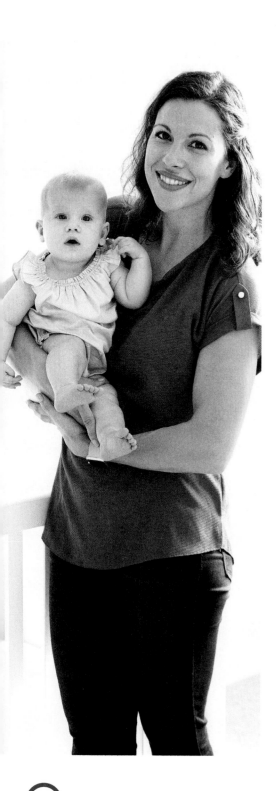

What is Happening to Your Body?

WHAT?

Whether you were discharged from the hospital within six hours or stayed a few nights, little prepares you for returning home with a baby. Your body is working overtime to heal, yet your baby will need you at all hours of the day and night, so clocking up sufficient rest will be a challenge.

Once you've survived the first couple weeks, your body will begin to feel a little more familiar. Mentally and emotionally, you're still in for a bit of a rollercoaster. Nothing will comfort your baby like closeness to you, which can feel as much of a burden as it is a blessing. Rest assured that this rollercoaster has many more ups than it has downs.

WHY?

Within a few days, your uterus will contract to its prenatal size. However, your stomach will remain squidgy for several more weeks. Be kind to that tummy – it has spent the last nine months stretching up to double its natural length and width. Your weakened core is also experiencing a number of new and unfamiliar demands. There's lifting and twisting to fit car seats and manoeuvre the pram, and postural challenges on your spine as you spend long hours nursing or soothing baby.

On the emotional front, pre-menstrual-like symptoms come from a dramatic drop in oestrogen and progesterone, accompanied by bleeding that can last up to two weeks as your body naturally sheds extra mucus and uterine tissue. It's not unusual for iron levels to be very low in the first month, which can go unnoticed as we often assume our fatigue is down to a newborn's capacity to sleep for just a few hours at a time.

SO WHAT?

First and foremost, be patient. Taking on too much, too fast is more likely to stall your body's recovery than it is to aid it. The majority of women experience some degree of diastasis recti – abdominal separation along the midline of the tummy – and it's important for this to heal slowly and safely in order to restore full functionality of the core muscles (see page 184).

If you breastfeed, your relaxin levels will remain high for several more months, meaning any joint instability you experienced during pregnancy will linger a while longer. Pair this instability with a substantially weakened pelvic floor and you will soon learn that minimising strain, impact and heavy lifting is essential throughout the fourth trimester.

Safeguard against iron deficiency by eating ample meat, or vegetarian sources such as beetroot and spinach. Now is the time to tuck into any meals you wisely froze ahead of baby's arrival. Ask visitors to come with healthy meals to support your recovery, and use both your loved ones and your network of doctors, midwives and health visitors to voice any concerns you have about your physical or mental well-being. If a slow return to training aids your sense of well-being, walking with baby or gentle exercise using a baby carrier can meet both your need for movement and baby's need for constant touch and comfort.

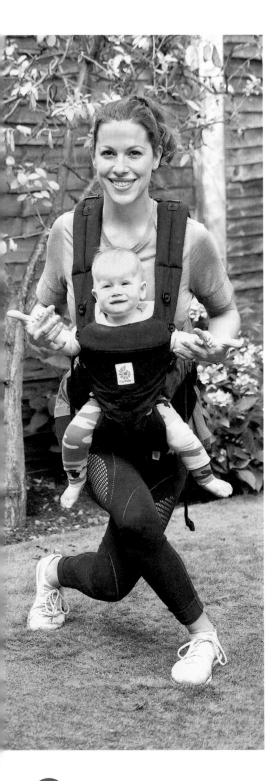

Postpartum Exercise

BENEFITS OF POSTPARTUM EXERCISE

Rest and exercise play equally important roles in your postpartum recovery. Here are just a few incentives to get back on your feet.

- Boosts blood flow to the perineum, aiding recovery of any stitching or tearing from a vaginal birth.

- Improves total body circulation, improving blood supply for breast milk production.

- Promotes the release of serotonin to counteract the effects of stress hormones and to aid postpartum hormonal stability.

- Encourages you to get outside and increase vitamin D absorption for both you and your newborn.

- Enhances emotional well-being by creating opportunities to socialise with others.

WHEN TO EASE OFF

Overexertion during your postpartum period can be very dangerous. A slow, steady recovery is always better than a sprint start with setbacks. Watch for the following symptoms of physical stress and remember to heal before you hurry.

BLEEDING HASN'T EASED OFF WITHIN TWO WEEKS OF BIRTH Consult your doctor if it remains heavy or becomes heavier.

YOU'RE LEAKING URINE DURING OR AFTER EXERCISE Prioritise your kegel exercises and bodyweight exercises with pelvic floor integration before adding load or impact.

THERE IS DOMING IN YOUR ABDOMINALS Your core is not yet strong enough to contain the intensity of intra-abdominal pressure. Regress your core exercises to avoid doming.

YOUR BACK HURTS Your core muscles are not supporting you through your choice of exercise. Regress the exercise and refocus on your glutes and deep-core activation.

YOU FEEL EXTREME FATIGUE As well as suffering from sleep deprivation, it is common to be slightly anaemic after childbirth. Stop training and focus on taking naps and getting sufficient iron through food or supplements. Consult your doctor if fatigue continues or worsens.

HOW TO CHECK FOR ABDOMINAL SEPARATION

Stretching of the abdominal muscles and fascia during pregnancy can cause separation along the linea alba (midline). This is simple to self-assess after birth, and it's important to do so as substantial separation (more than two fingers) requires careful core function rehabilitation to aid your posture, support your organs and prevent greater trouble such as a lower back injury or hernia.

1. Lie on your back with your feet planted and your spine in neutral. Cushion your head with one hand, keeping the elbow wide.
2. Press firmly with two fingers just above your navel, palm facing you.
3. Lift your shoulders from the floor and draw your chin towards your chest. You should feel two slightly elevated sides of your rectus abdominis.
4. If there is more than a two-finger width separation between these two sides, take special care to avoid crunching movements. This means rolling on to your side and using your hands for support when moving from lying to seated or standing. Use the Core Restore progressions (see page 184) before advancing your abs exercises.
5. For a more in-depth pelvic floor and core function analysis, book an appointment with a women's health physiotherapist.

Beginnings & Endings

Your return to exercise begins here. Once your uterus has fully contracted, you can comfortably walk for more than half an hour at a time and you are coping with the physical demands of life with your newborn, you can begin to introduce gentle movement into your day. The following movements and stretches are great to practise while baby enjoys daily tummy time. Moving together is bonding together. Use these movements in isolation or as a warm-up and cool-down once you're ready for more structured workouts.

POSTPARTUM WARM-UP

Try to incorporate each of the following movements several times a day, whenever you have a convenient moment while baby plays or naps. Complete two circuits if incorporating as a warm-up to further exercise.

KEGELS

Build up to ten slow squeezes, holding each for five to ten seconds, followed by ten to twenty fast squeezes. Remember to relax your glutes and think about lifting the pelvic floor from back to front, finishing with the 'belt-tightening' engagement of your deep-core muscles.

TIP: Kegel exercises are even more useful postnatally than they are prenatally, as they are essential to both the healing process and re-strengthening the muscles fundamental to everyday movement and structured exercise. Start as soon as you can after birth and incorporate them frequently – ideally eight times a day. Try doing them while you nurse or bottlefeed your baby to build them into your routine.

PELVIC TILTS

1. Lie with your back on the floor, your spine in neutral and your feet planted.
2. Slowly draw your navel down and flatten your back to the floor by gently scooping up your hips. Think about magnetising your pubic bone towards your rib cage.
3. Avoid putting pressure into your feet – this movement should come from your deep core, not your glutes. Work through ten slow reps.

RECLINE RAINBOWS

1. From an upright, seated position, lean back ten to thirty degrees until you feel a gentle awakening in your tummy. You can rest your hands on the outside of your knees for extra support.
2. From recline, find your C-curve position on the exhale, thinking about magnetising pubic bone and rib cage.
3. Hold for a moment, then reverse on the inhale and gently arch your spine as you press your belly towards your thighs. It may feel nice to stretch your arms overhead to increase the stretch in your chest.
4. Work through ten slow, breath-accompanied spinal rolls.

ECCENTRIC SQUAT

1. Eccentric squats are a powerful way to strengthen overstretched iliopsoas hip flexors. Stand with your back to a seat that is roughly knee height or higher. Slowly descend to a seated position, moving no faster than a count of five.
2. Return to standing for a count of one, exhaling and engaging your pelvic floor as you do so. Build up to ten reps.

POSTPARTUM COOL-DOWN

Incorporate these stretches throughout the day as necessary, or work through them once consecutively for fifteen to sixty seconds as instructed to encourage optimal mobility post-workout.

SUPPORTED PUPPY STRETCH

1. Rest your hands on an elevated platform, shuffling your body back until your hips are square over your knees and your arms are straight. Now allow your chest to soften towards the floor, feeling the stretch across your upper back.
2. This is a lovely stretch to hold through a few breath cycles, or to make dynamic by rolling the spine away from the floor on the exhale and softening the chest towards the floor on the inhale.

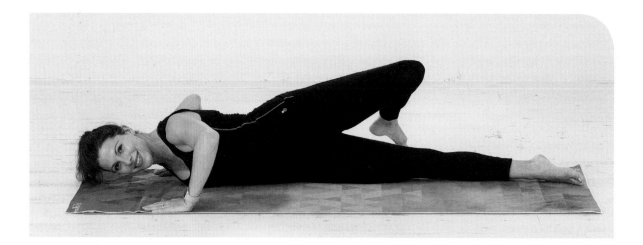

COBRA STRETCH

1. Lie on your tummy with your hands by your chest.
2. Without using momentum, gently push your pubic bone down, draw your navel in and lift your shoulders away from the floor. You can use your fingertips to support you at the top of the lift.
3. Hold here for five breath cycles, or alternately rotate and gaze over one shoulder at a time for ten repetitions.

SCORPION STRETCH

1. Lie on your tummy with your arms parallel and your chest gently lifted.
2. Bend one foot to the sky and open through the hip as you tap the toe to the floor behind the other knee (shown above).
3. Return to centre and repeat to the other side for a total of ten reps, exhaling with the twist.

SIDE-LYING THORACIC OPENER

1. Lie on your side with your knees stacked and slightly bent, and your arms extended with your palms touching.
2. Lift your top arm up and around in a big circle until the back of your palm reaches the floor behind you. Allow your hip to open gently as required.
3. Open on the inhale and close on the exhale, repeating for five to ten reps before switching sides.

LYING LEG TWIST

1. Lie on your back and draw your knees into your chest.
2. Gently allow your knees to fall to the floor on one side, simultaneously encouraging the opposite shoulder to remain grounded.
3. Breathe into your lower back. Use each exhale to deepen the stretch, holding for up to sixty seconds before switching sides to repeat.

HAMSTRING & PIRIFORMIS STRETCH

1. Lying on your back with your legs long, draw one leg up to the ceiling and wrap a resistance band around the foot so you have equal tension on the band in each hand.
2. Flex your foot and gently draw your toe towards your nose while sending your tailbone down. Hold for five breath cycles.
3. Now transfer both ends of the band into your inside hand and gently pull the straight leg a few centimetres towards the resting leg. You should feel a deep stretch down the IT band. Hold for five breath cycles.
4. Repeat both of the above on the opposite leg.

KNEELING HIP-FLEXOR STRETCH

1. Kneel on one leg and plant the other foot in front, checking the heel is in line with the back knee and the hips are level. You can support your hand using a yoga block or upright foam roller outside the front leg to help maintain a neutral pelvis.
2. Now send the pubic bone forwards until you feel a stretch through the front and side of the back hip – focus on the area where the top outside corner of your jeans pocket sits.
3. Hold for up to sixty seconds before switching sides – the longer the better to encourage these overworked muscles to 'remember' the stretch.

Core Restore

The abdominal muscles are understandably weakened and lengthened after birth. But it's too early to jump back into traditional abs-toning moves just now. Most women will experience some separation along the midline of the stomach, and if it hasn't happened during pregnancy it can happen as a result of excess intra-abdominal pressure during the postpartum recovery. These separation-safe exercises will help you knit the muscles back together and strengthen the underlying core muscles so you can soon make a safe and strong return to all your favourite exercises.

Use the following exercises as consecutive progressions, building up to performing all four in one routine only once you're confident with the preceding exercise(s). With each, think about drawing your tummy muscles down and in. Feel or watch your stomach and check that there's no doming around the midline of your abdominals.

PELVIC TILT WITH SLOW KEGELS

1. Lie on your back with a neutral spine and your heels gently planted.
2. As you curl the base of your spine off the floor, squeeze your pelvic floor muscles without clenching your glutes. Hold the squeeze for up to ten seconds. Build up to ten reps.

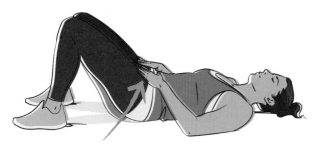

CAT COW WITH FAST KEGELS

1. Kneel on all fours, maintaining a soft bend in your elbows.
2. When you hit the top of your cat pose, scoop your abdominal muscles in and simultaneously squeeze your pelvic floor muscles in three quick successive pulses, accompanied with short successive exhales.
3. Relax your pelvic floor as you inhale to cow pose. Build up to ten reps.

HEEL SLIDES

1. Lie on your back with a neutral spine and your heels gently planted.
2. Ensure there is no strain on your lower back as you slowly extend one heel at a time along the floor.
3. Think about maintaining the natural arch of your spine so that you're pulling the abdominals together but not forcing your lumbar to the floor. Exhale and engage the pelvic floor with each extension. Build up to twenty alternating reps.

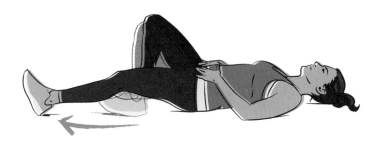

PLANK SHIFTERS

1. Come to a forearm down-dog position with palms upturned to help prevent excess load in the shoulders. Inhale and relax your abdominals.
2. On the exhale, lower the knees, tuck the hips and scoop the midsection to your half plank position. Look for a gentle quiver in the abs as you connect all the components of the core, but don't hold through intense shaking. Gradually build to ten reps with ten second holds.

ALL-FOURS HOVERS

1. Use all fours as an active recovery, drawing your tummy muscles inwards as your spine sits parallel to the floor.
2. Tuck your toes and elevate your knees, keeping that active tension in your stomach muscles without strain or doming. Gradually build up to ten reps with ten second holds.

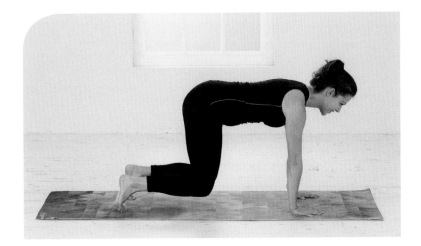

Baby Bonding & Strength Building

This workout is all about enjoying more structured exercise by bonding with your newborn and using baby for added resistance. Early in the fourth trimester babies can only see a metre in distance and will crave visual and physical closeness. By carrying your baby in a sling while exercising, you'll meet both its needs and yours. If you're not comfortable wearing your baby in a sling, you can substitute a light kettlebell for these exercises.

Work through ten to fifteen reps of each exercise and two to four sets of each circuit, prioritising optimal form and gradually adding reps and sets as you get stronger. Make sure you're confident in the safe babywearing guidelines specific to your babycarrier. Babies should face in until six months and you should observe the universal TICKS check: baby is positioned **t**ightly, **i**n sight, **c**lose enough to kiss, chin **k**ept off the chest and their back **s**upported.

Equipment

Light kettlebell
(4–8kg /9–18lb)

Resistance band

CIRCUIT ONE

SPLIT SQUATS
—

1. Place one foot about 1m (3ft) in front of the chair and rest the back forefoot on the edge of the seat. Absorb your weight in the front foot.
2. Bend through the front knee until your thigh is just above parallel with the floor. Check the knee is stacked over the heel and the weight remains in the heel.
3. Push through the heel to return to standing. Do all your reps on one side before switching. Stay close to a wall or use extra support if you feel unbalanced.

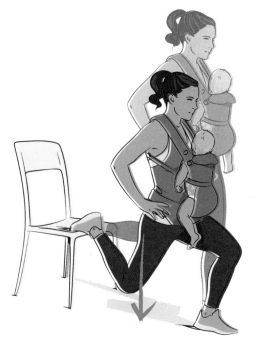

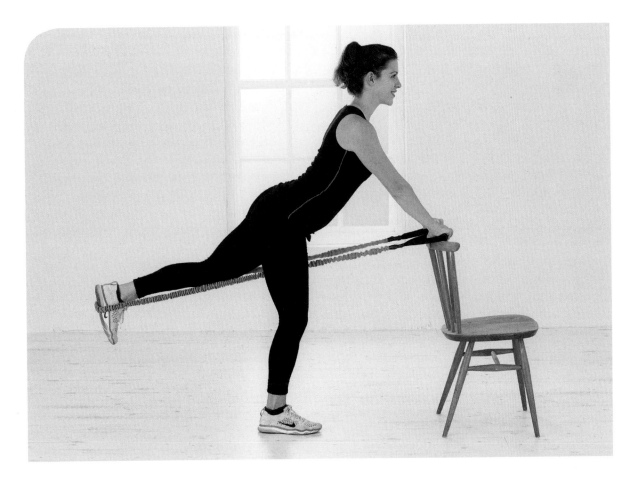

STANDING BANDED KICKBACKS

1. Standing behind the chair, anchor both ends of a resistance band under your palms on the back of the chair and loop the centre around one heel.
2. Maintain a soft bend in the standing leg as you draw the other knee towards your navel then squeeze the back of the leg and the glutes to extend the leg straight back.
3. Do all your reps on one side before switching.

CURTSY LUNGES

1. Standing alongside the chair for optional support, absorb your weight in your outside leg as you bend your inside knee back and behind the standing leg.
2. Push through the heel to return to standing and draw your inside knee towards your navel, simultaneously engaging the pelvic floor and tightening your deep core.
3. Do all your reps on one side before switching.

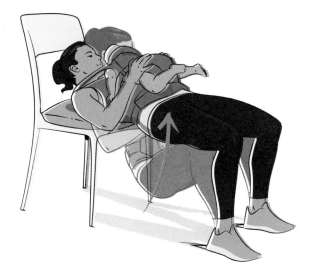

ELEVATED HIP THRUSTS

1. Make sure the seat of the chair is well cushioned. Rest your mid-back against the edge of the seat and plant both feet firmly on the floor.
2. Pivoting along your bra line, lower your hips below knee level then squeeze your glutes to lift your hips back in line with your heart. Your baby should now be in full prone position against your chest.

Modification: If this feels easy, shuffle one foot a few centimetres into centre and try a single-leg variation.

CIRCUIT TWO

CHAIR-ANCHORED SHOULDER OPENERS

1. Stand 30–60cm (1–2ft) away from the chair and rest one foot on the seat to hold it in place; wrap a resistance band around the back of the chair and hold the ends with equal tension in both hands.
2. Engage your core to stabilise your trunk and draw your shoulders together as you pull your arms behind you with straight elbows. You should feel the work in your lats running down the sides of your back.

CHAIR-ANCHORED SERVING PLATTERS

1. Start in the same position as above, switching the elevated leg.
2. Turn your palms up and hug your elbows into your waist. Without moving your elbows, open your forearms out to the sides until your hands are in line with your rib cage. Feel the squeeze between your shoulders and the stretch across your chest.

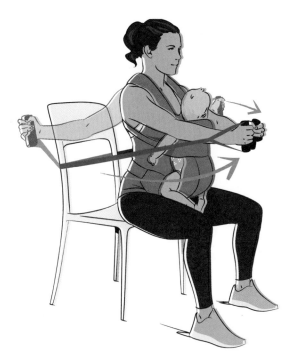

CHAIR CHEST FLIES

1. Sit on the chair with the ends of the band in each hand and the centre of it wrapped around the back of the chair.
2. Scoot as far forward in the seat as you need to feel tension in the band as you extend your arms to the sides.
3. Engage your core and exhale as you draw your palms together. Pause through centre and inhale to return to the start.

SEATED TRICEP EXTENSIONS

1. Set up as per the previous exercise, but turn your palms to face one another and frame your elbows around your chest with your hands just above your shoulders.
2. Keep wrapping your elbows in as you extend your arms. Don't let your elbows flare out or drop below your chest.

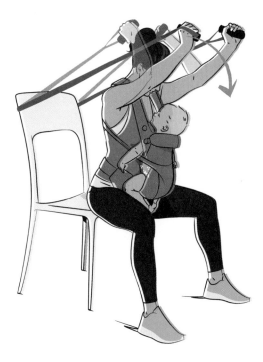

Index

Sources

In order of reference:

Maternal and fetal development updates appearing throughout *Mind, Body, Bump* are sourced from a combination of public health support materials published by the NHS, Tommy's and BabyCentre.

O'Connor, Poudevigne, Cress, Motl, Clapp, '**Safety and Efficacy of Supervised Strength Training Adopted in Pregnancy**', *Journal of Physical Activity and Health*, March 2011

Federation of American Societies for Experimental Biology, '**Labor of love: Physically active moms-to-be give babies a head start on heart health**', *Science Daily*, August 2011

Newcomer, Bahls, Sheldon, Taheripour, Clifford, Foust, Breslin, Marchant-Forde, Cabot, Laughlin, Bidwell, '**Exercise during pregnancy improves vascular function of offspring into adulthood**', *Journal of Experimental Physiology*, October 2013

Kardel, Johansen, Voldner, Iversen, Henriksen, '**Association between aerobic fitness in late pregnancy and duration of labor in nulliparous women**', *Scandinavian Journal of Obstetrics and Gynaecology*, 2009

Kahyaoglu Sut H, Balkanli Kaplan P, '**Effect of Pelvic Floor Muscle Exercise on Pelvic Floor Muscle Activity and Voiding Functions During Pregnancy and the Postpartum Period**', *The Cochrane Collaboration*, Issue 12, 2017

Labonte-LeMoyne, University of Montreal, '**Exercise during pregnancy enhances a newborn's brain development**', findings shared at Neuroscience 2013 congress in San Diego

Kardel, '**Effects of Intense Training During and After Pregnancy in Top-Level Athletes**', *Scandinavian Journal of Medical Science & Sports*, April 2005

Stutzman, Brown, Hains, Godwin, Smith, Parlow, '**Effects of Exercise Conditioning in Normal and Overweight Pregnant Women in Blood Pressure and Heart Rate Variability**', *Biological Research in Nursing*, Issue 12, 2010

Howard, Ryan, Trevillion, Anderson, '**Accuracy of the Whooley questions and the Edinburgh Postnatal Depression Scale in identifying depression and other mental disorders in pregnancy**', *British Journal of Psychiatry*, January 2018

Mennella, Jagnow, Beauchamp, '**Prenatal and Postnatal Flavor Learning by Human Infants**', *Journal of Pediatrics*, June 2001

Newham, Wittkowski, Hurley, Aplin, Westwood, '**Effects of Antenatal Yoga on Maternal Anxiety and Depression**', *Depression and Anxiety Journal*, April 2014

Raymann, Swaab, Van Someren, '**Skin Deep: Enhanced Sleep Depth by Cutaneous Temperature Manipulation**', *Brain Journal*, February 2008

Sun-Edelstein, Mauskop, '**Alternative headache treatments**', *Headache Journal*, February 2011

Bath, Hill, Goenaga Infante, Elghul, Nezianya, Rayman, '**Iodine concentration of milk-alternative drinks available in the UK in comparison with cows' milk**', *British Journal of Nutrition*, 2017

Kordi, Meyodi, Tara, Nemati, Taghi-Shakeri, '**The Effect of Late Pregnancy Consumption of Date Fruit**', *Journal of Midwifery and Reproductive Health*, July 2014

Acknowledgements

Dedicated to the bumps who teach us to love our bodies.

Thank you to Philippa, Kerry & Emma at White Lion Publishing and Jane at Graham Maw Christie Literary Agency for seeing the potential in an idea and sharing in the vision that has brought it to life.

Thank you to consultant obstetrician Dr Maggie Blott, who knows the prenatal body better than any other, and whose diligence in reviewing *Mind, Body, Bump* for medical accuracy has vastly enriched these pages.

Thank you to Tamara, who believed in *empowered women* and *active motherhood* long before they became hashtags, and who was the first and only person I envisioned writing the foreword to this book.

Thank you to the strong women in my life who inspire me every day. To my clients who give me their trust and friendship at the squat rack. To my peers in the fitness industry who believe that sharing, not comparing, is the key to growing stronger together. To my closest friends who encouraged me to take stock of this milestone and celebrate the mini-victories in its creation.

Thank you to my parents, who supported every unexpected turn in my career and gave me space to do things differently.

Thank you to my husband Ben, who never questioned my optimism (read: insanity) in signing a book deal days before the birth of our daughter, and who selflessly committed to the task of keeping me sane through the subsequent months of juggling diapers and deadlines.

Which brings me to the bump – now the baby. Thank you to Marnie, whose existence gave life to the idea for *Mind, Body, Bump*. In sharing my body, you taught me to respect and nurture it more than ever before.